100 No-Equipment Workouts

Volume 3

2019

N. Rey | darebee.com

First Printing, 2019.
ISBN 13: 978-1-84481-014-7
ISBN 10: 1-84481-014-3

Warning and Disclaimer
Although every precaution has been taken to verify the accuracy of
the information contained herein, the author and publisher assume no responsibility for any errors or
omissions. No liability is assumed for damage or injury that may result from the use of information
contained within.

100 workouts - Volume III

1. 100 Push-Ups
2. Action Time
3. Ankle Recovery
4. Antihero
5. Ants in My Pants
6. Anywhere Cardio
7. Back to Basics
8. Beer Belly
9. Bubble Butt
10. Burn & Build
11. Busy Bee
12. Cardio & Core Burn
13. Cardio Fix
14. Chopper
15. Coda
16. Combat HIIT
17. Core Twister
18. Critical Hit
19. Crushing It!
20. Cyberpunk
21. Deathsquad
22. Defiant
23. Do Over
24. Expedited Delivery
25. Extra Spice
26. Fab Abs
27. Feel Good
28. Femme Fatale
29. Fresh Start
30. Genesis
31. Get It Done
32. Good Morning Yoga
33. Grit & Grace
34. Gut
35. Hello, abs!
36. Hero
37. Hip Dips
38. Holistic
39. Homemade Abs
40. Homemade Hero
41. Huff & Puff
42. Inquisitor
43. Into The Fire
44. Lady Knight
45. Lean & Mean
46. Live Long
47. Lunch
48. Make My Day
49. Micro Shred
50. Monkey!
51. Monster Inside
52. Morning Stretch
53. Nix
54. No Surrender
55. Odyssey
56. Off Day
57. One-Minute
58. Onna Bugeisha
59. Outlaw
60. Overkill
61. Over The Rainbow
62. Pack A Punch
63. Party Time
64. Permission Granted
65. Player
66. Pouncer
67. Powerbuilt
68. Power Burner
69. Power Gainer
70. Pump & Burn
71. Quick HIIT
72. Rambler
73. Rascal
74. Ravager
75. Raw Grit
76. Reconstructor
77. Rectifier
78. Red Reaper
79. Rest & Rec
80. Reviver
81. Rewired
82. Ricochet
83. Rockin' Abs
84. Rogue Build
85. Siren
86. Skybreaker
87. Storm
88. Strongman
89. Super Burn
90. Superhero Abs
91. Super HIIT
92. Superhuman
93. Sweat Zone
94. Target Abs
95. Ultimatum
96. Upperbody Tendons
97. Upperbody Works
98. Walk, Run, Repeat
99. White Rabbit
100. Zone

Introduction

Bodyweight training may look easy, but if you are not used to it, it's very far from that. It is just as intense as running and it is just as challenging so if you struggle with it at the very beginning, it's perfectly ok – you will get better at it once you start doing it regularly. Do it at your own pace and take longer breaks if you need to.

You can start with a single individual workout from the collection and see how you feel. If you are new to bodyweight training always start any workout on Level I (level of difficulty).

You can pick any number of workouts per week, usually between 3 and 5 and rotate them for maximum results.

Some workouts are more suitable for weight loss and toning up and others are more strength oriented, some do both. To make it easier for you to choose, they have all been labelled according to FOCUS, use it to design a training regimen based on your goal.

High Burn and Strength oriented workouts will help you with your weight, aerobic capacity and muscle tone, some are just more specialized, but it doesn't mean you should exclusively focus on one or the other. Whatever your goal with bodyweight training you'll benefit from doing exercises that produce results in both areas.

This collection has been designed to be completely no-equipment for maximum accessibility so several bodyweight exercises like pull-ups have been excluded. If you want to work on your biceps and back more and you have access to a pull-up bar, have one at home or can use it somewhere else like the nearest playground (monkey bars), you can do wide and close grip pull-ups, 3 sets to failure 2-3 times a week with up to 2 minutes rest in between sets in addition to your training. Alternatively, you can add pull-ups at the beginning or at the end of every set of a Strength Oriented workout.

All of the routines in this collection are suitable for both men and women, no age restrictions apply.

The Manual

Workout posters are read from left to right and contain the following information: grid with exercises (images), number of reps (repetitions) next to each, number of sets for your fitness level (I, II or III) and rest time.

SAMPLE WORKOUT

LEVEL I 3 sets LEVEL II 5 sets LEVEL III 7 sets REST up to 2 minutes

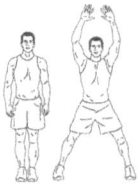

10 jumping jacks

20 high knees

40 side-to-side chops

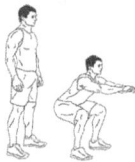

10 squats

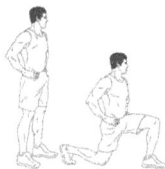

20 lunges

10-count plank

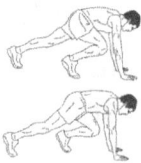

20 climbers

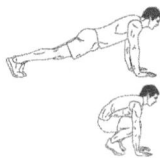

10 plank jump-ins

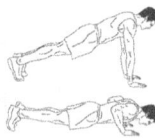

to failure push-ups

Difficulty Levels:

Level I: normal

Level II: hard

Level III: advanced

1 set

10 jumping jacks

20 high knees (10 each leg)

40 side-to-side chops (20 each side)

10 squats

20 lunges (10 each leg)

10-count plank (hold while counting to 10)

20 climbers (10 each leg)

10 plank jump-ins

to failure push-ups (your maximum)

Up to 2 minutes rest between sets

30 seconds, 60 seconds or 2 minutes - it's up to you.

"Reps" stands for repetitions, how many times an exercise is performed. Reps are usually located next to each exercise's name. Number of reps is always a total number for both legs / arms / sides. It's easier to count this way: e.g. if it says 20 climbers, it means that both legs are already counted in - it is 10 reps each leg.

Reps to failure means to muscle failure = your personal maximum, you repeat the move until you can't. It can be anything from one rep to twenty, normally applies to more challenging exercises. The goal is to do as many as you possibly can.

The transition from exercise to exercise is an important part of each circuit (set) - it is often what makes a particular workout more effective. Transitions are carefully worked out to hyperload specific muscle groups more for better results. For example if you see a plank followed by push-ups it means that you start performing push-ups right after you finished with the plank avoiding dropping your body on the floor in between.

There is no rest between exercises - only after sets, unless specified otherwise. You have to complete the entire set going from one exercise to the next as fast as you can before you can rest.

What does "up to 2 minutes rest" mean: it means you can rest for up to 2 minutes but the sooner you can go again the better. Eventually your recovery time will improve naturally, you won't need all two minutes to recover - and that will also be an indication of your improving fitness.

Recommended rest time:

Level I: 2 minutes or less
Level II: 60 seconds or less
Level III: 30 seconds or less

If you can't do all out push-ups yet on Level I it is perfectly acceptable to do knee push-ups instead. The modification works the same muscles as a full push-up but lowers the load significantly helping you build up on it first. It is also ok to switch to knee push-ups at any point if you can no longer do full push-ups in the following sets.

Video Exercise Library
http://darebee.com/video

The workouts are organized in alphabetical order so you can find the workouts you favor easier and faster.

1 100 Push-Ups

A 100 push-up routine is the core of this combat moves and core workout. Push-ups are a great total-body exercise routine, by dressing it up with exercises that demand both eccentric and concentric muscle movements we end up with a workout that's worthy of every warrior.

Focus: Upperbody Strength

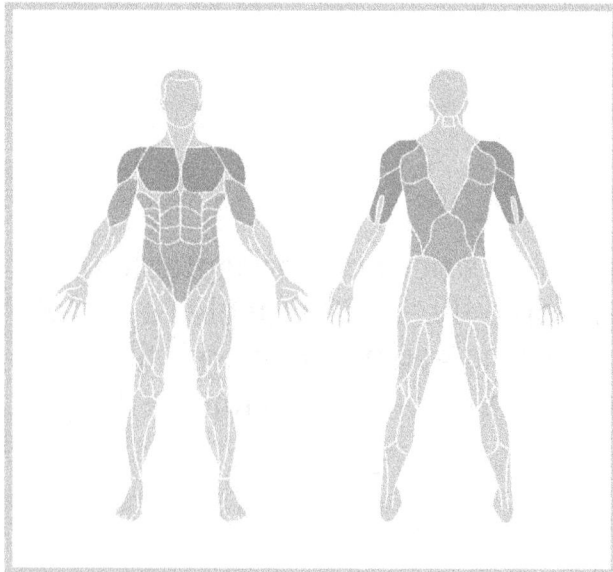

100 PUSH-UPS

DAREBEE WORKOUT © darebee.com

Repeat 5 times in total   2 minutes rest between sets

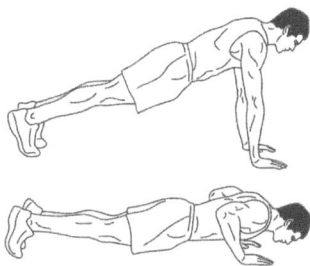

5 push-ups

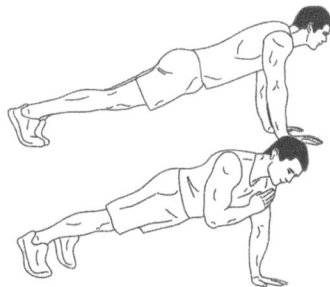

20 shoulder taps

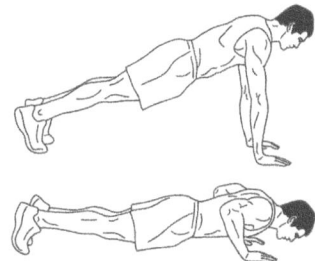

5 push-ups

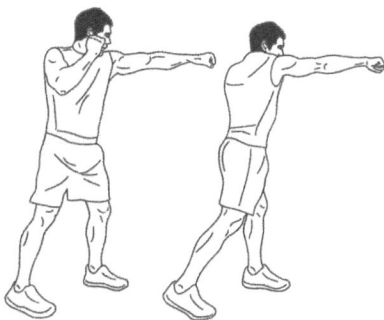

20 punches

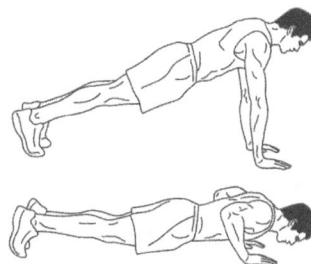

10 push-ups

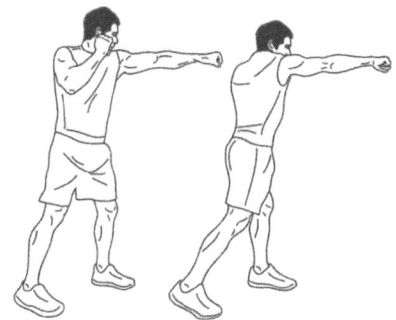

20 punches

2 Action Time

Action Time Workout is, essentially, a supercharged burpee but with double the pain you get double the benefits. Keep your body straight during planks and don't drop down during planks and their transitions. Your ultimate goal is to keep the plank throughout never dropping down to your knees... even though you will really, really want to.

Focus: High Burn

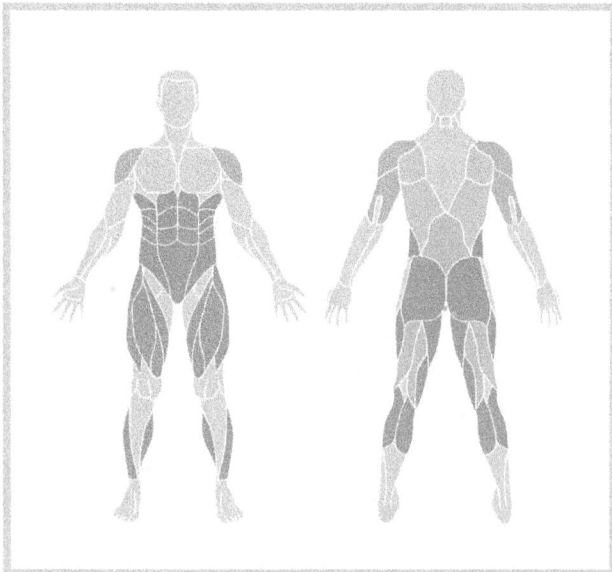

ACTION TIME

DAREBEE HIIT WORKOUT © darebee.com

Level I 3 sets **Level II** 5 sets **Level III** 7 sets | 2 minutes rest

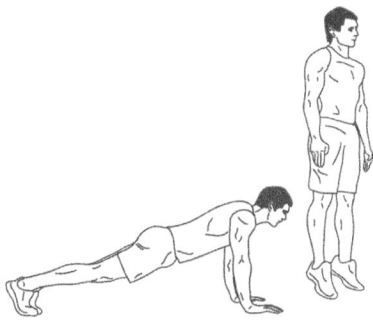

20sec basic burpees

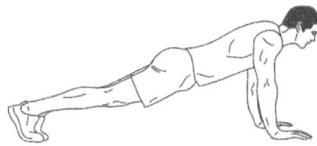

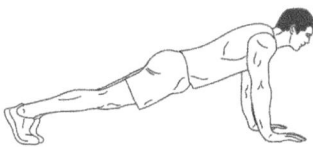

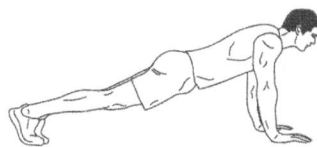

20sec plank hold

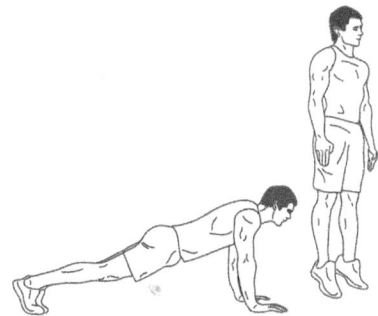

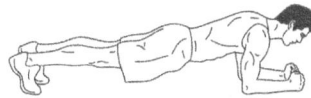

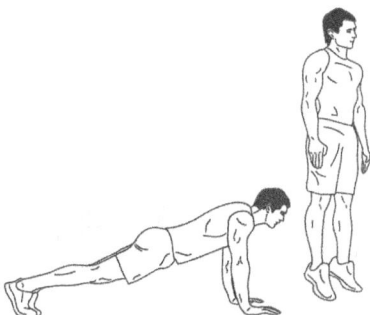

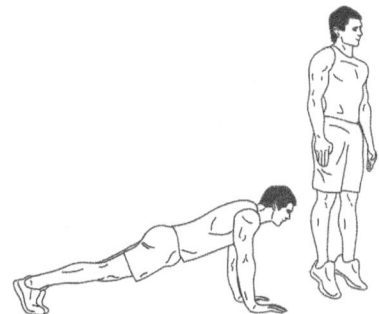

20sec basic burpees

20sec plank hold

20sec elbow plank hold

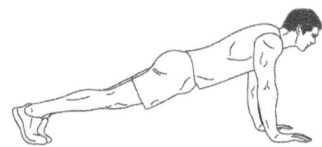

20sec plank hold

20sec basic burpees

20sec plank hold

20sec basic burpees

3   Ankle Recovery

Ankles are the overlooked joint. Because we can't flex it like biceps or feel that it contributes to our sense of power like quads do, we tend to think about it only when it goes wrong and then we realize that we can't run, can't kick, can't jump and, because our legs cannot work properly, we cannot even punch. Ankle Recovery remedies this by giving you a set of exercises to do that will help an injured ankle get better, faster plus this is a great workout to use as a preventative measure by incorporating it in any of your regular workouts.

Focus: Rehab

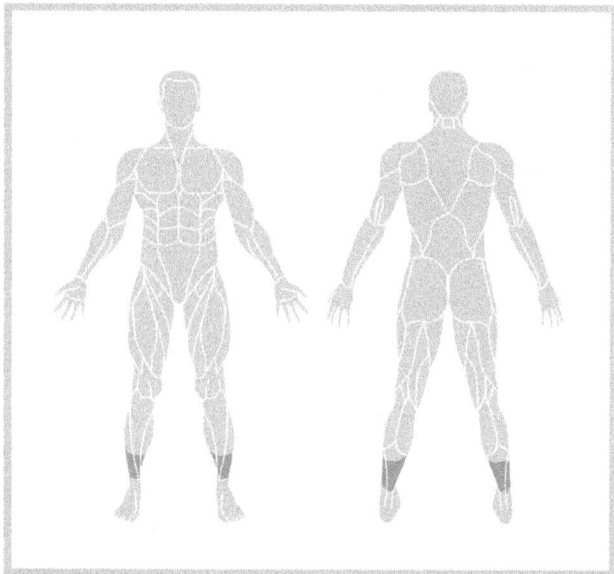

ankle
recovery

DAREBEE WORKOUT © darebee.com
30 seconds each exercise.

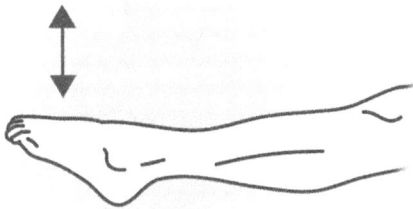

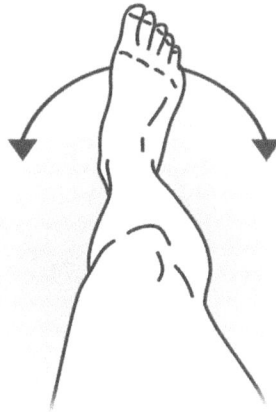

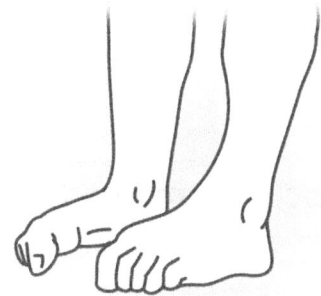

up and down tilts

side-to-side tilts

toe curls

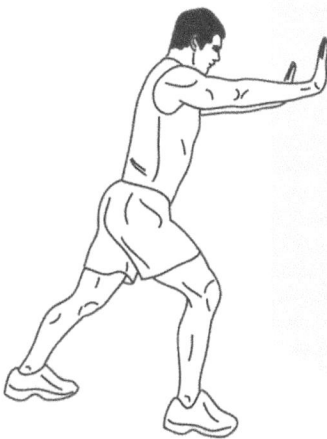

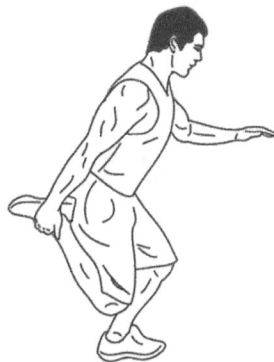

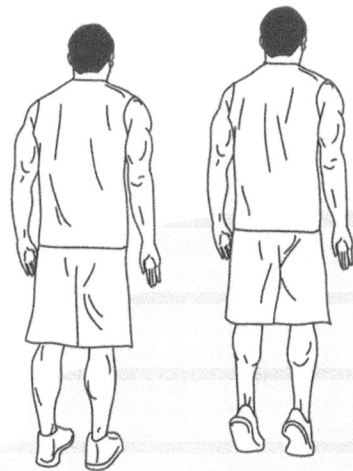

calf stretch

single leg balance

elevated calf raises

4   Antihero

Ironically being an anti-hero requires way more work than being a hero (and there is no cape to go with the description). That's because you need to stay up to scratch on your own. Without radioactive spiders willing to bite you, gammar ray experiments to sub-cellularly alter you or a red sun to affect your molecular structure you have to be more than enough under your own capabilities. That means hard work and the Antihero workout delivers that in spades.

Focus: Strength & Tone

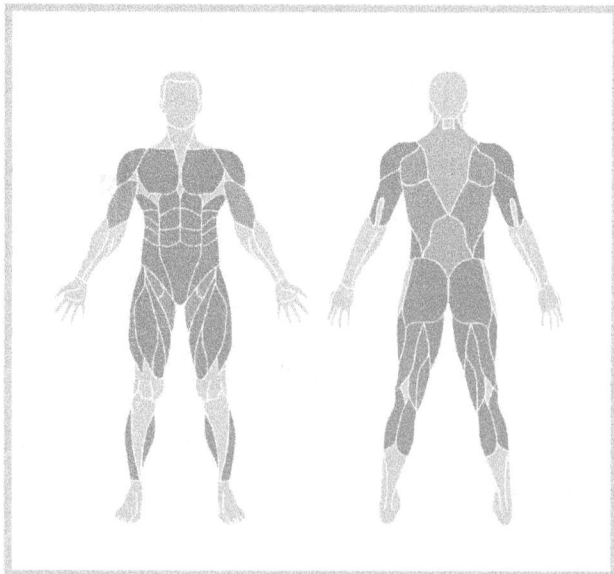

ANTIHERO

DAREBEE WORKOUT © darebee.com

LEVEL I 3 sets **LEVEL II** 5 sets **LEVEL III** 7 sets **REST** up to 2 minutes

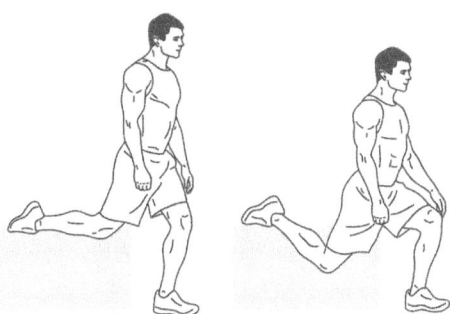

20 split squats

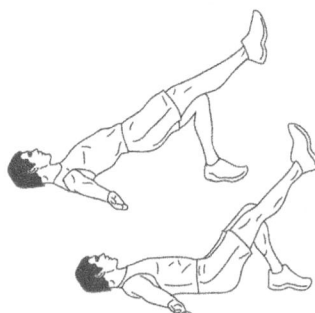

20 single leg bridges

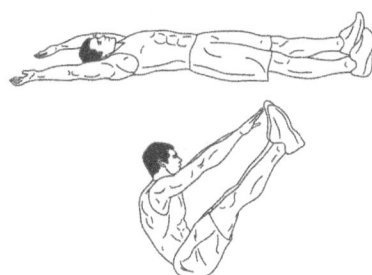

20 V-ups

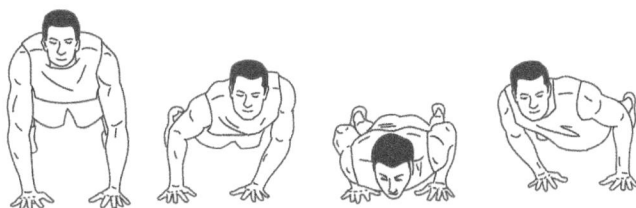

10 circle push-ups

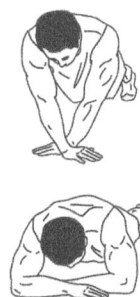

10 cross tricep extensions

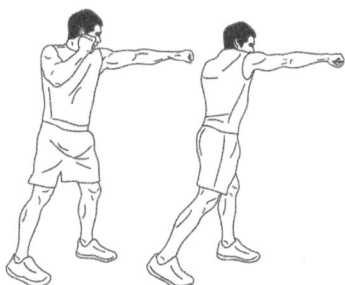

40 punches

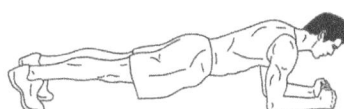

40sec elbow plank hold

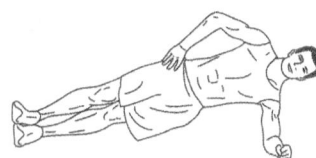

40sec side elbow plank

5   Ants in My Pants

Ants In My Pants lives up to its billing because you literally have zero downtime here. With exercises that flow from standing up to floor and back the workout uses Jumping Jacks to jack-up the pressure pushing not just your calf muscles to the limit but also your VO2 Max. Remember your heels never touch down during Jumping Jacks and your fingertips meet at the apex point over your head. Master it!

Focus: High Burn

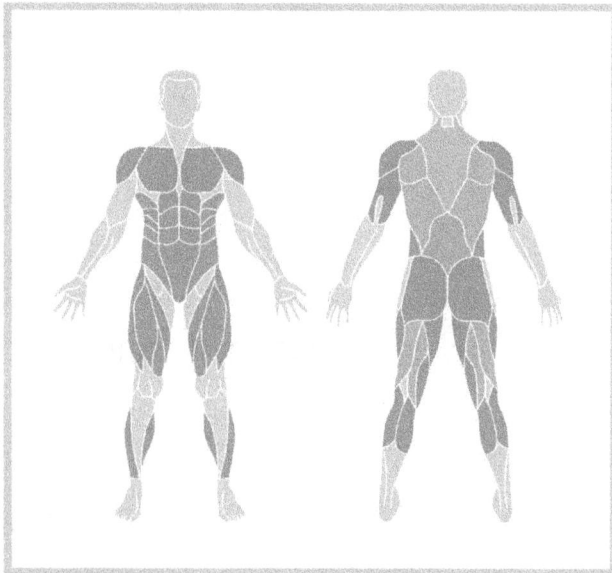

Ants in My Pants

DAREBEE `HIIT` WORKOUT © darebee.com

Level I 3 sets **Level II** 5 sets **Level III** 7 sets | 2 minutes rest

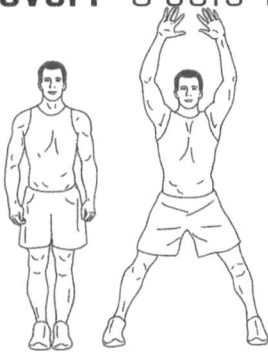

20sec jumping jacks

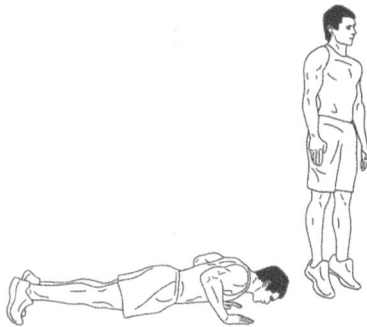

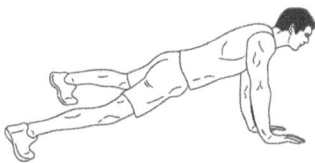

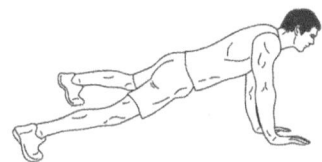

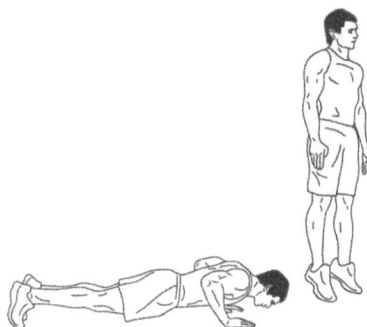

20sec burpees

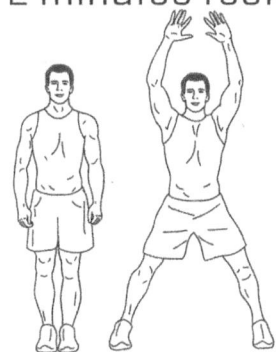

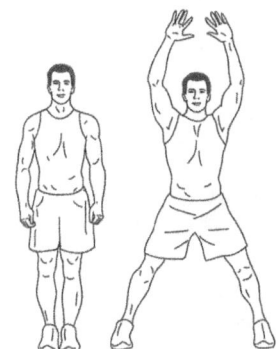

20sec jumping jacks

20sec wide plank hold

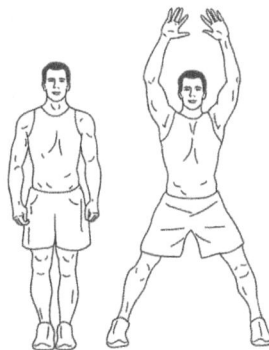

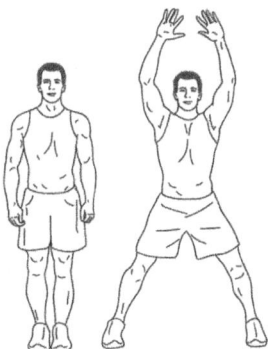

20sec jumping jacks

20sec wide plank hold

20sec jumping jacks

20sec burpees

20sec jumping jacks

6   Anywhere Cardio

You need, maybe a couple of minutes in total and a tiny space to stand and you have got yourself an awesome cardiovascular workout that will get your body going and your heart revving. Anywhere Cardio is a light, fast workout that's perfect for those times when time, space and even focus are in short supply. Have it on your horizon and you will never be stuck for a workout when the odds are against you.

Focus: High Burn

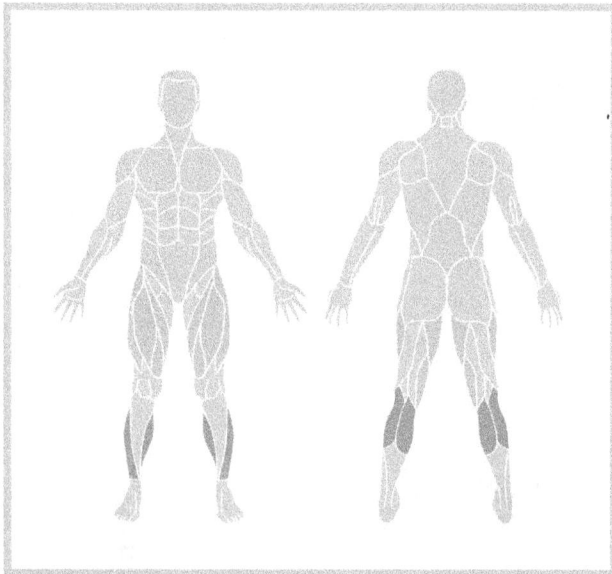

anywhere
cardio

DAREBEE WORKOUT © darebee.com

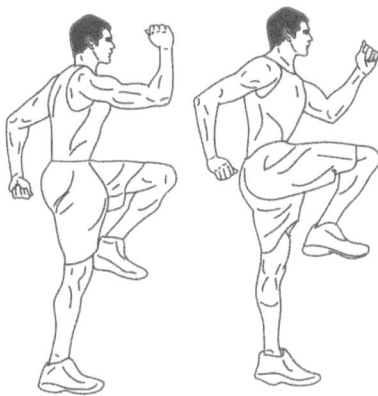

40 march steps **x 4 sets** in total
20 seconds rest in between sets

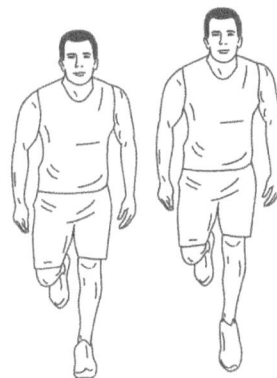

40 hops on the spot **x 2 sets** in total
no rest between sets 1 set per leg

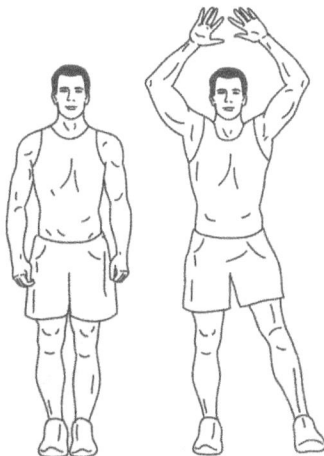

40 side jacks **x 4 sets** in total
20 seconds rest in between sets

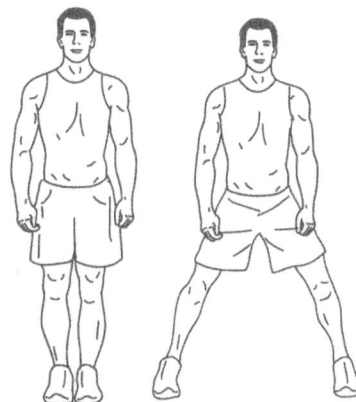

40 half jacks **x 4 sets** in total
20 seconds rest in between sets

7 Back to Basics

Basic training provides a firm foundation upon which we can build a stronger, fitter physique. Back to Basics is a workout that is, to all appearances, easy. Yet it works a large number of satellite muscle groups that engage when we are performing complex athletic moves. By raising the bar at this very basic level, this is the workout you need to turn to when you're contemplating getting fitter and you ask, "How can I start?"

Focus: High Burn

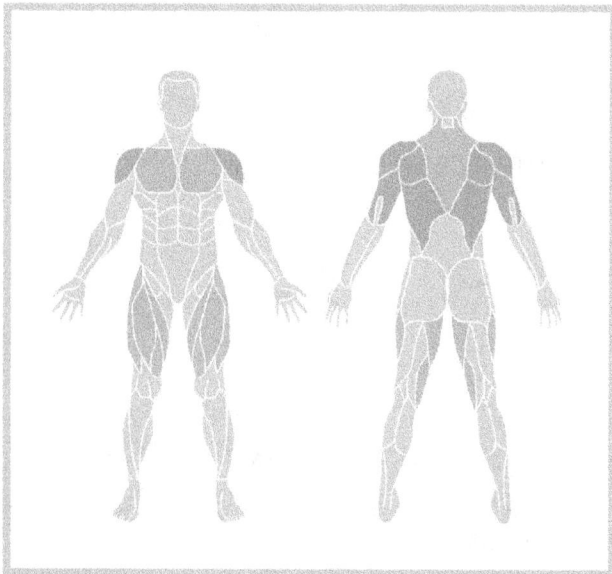

Back to Basics

DAREBEE WORKOUT © darebee.com

LEVEL I 3 sets **LEVEL II** 5 sets **LEVEL III** 7 sets **REST** up to 2 minutes

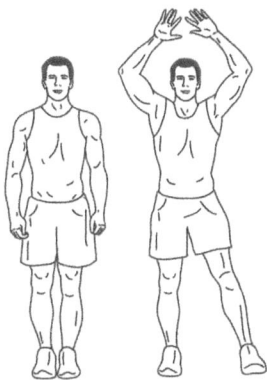

20 step jacks

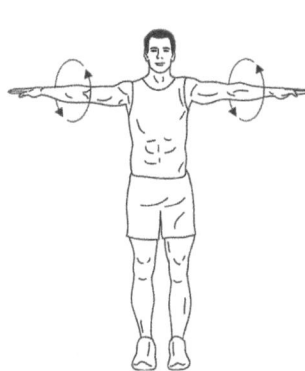

20 raised arm circles

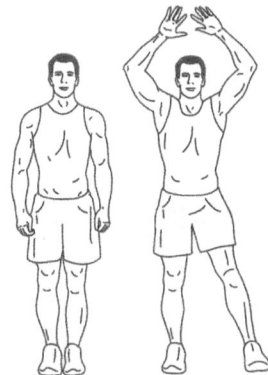

20 step jacks

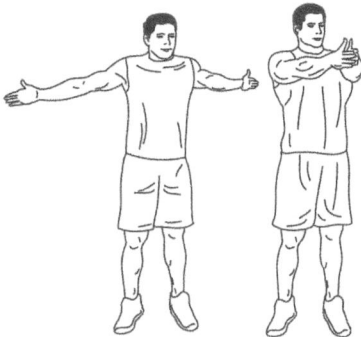

20 chest expansions

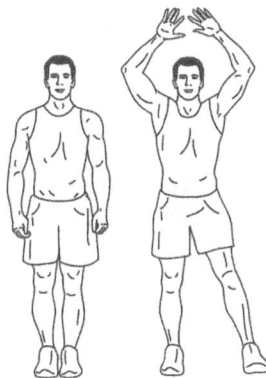

20 step jacks

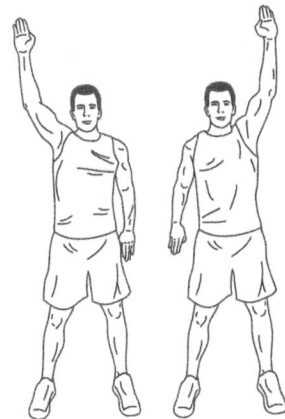

20 alt chest expansions

8 Beer Belly

While there is no workout routine, set of exercises or program that will allow you to lose weight locally, there are exercise routines that will tighten your abs, work your core and raise your body temperature putting you, squarely, in the sweatzone. The Beer Belly workout is one of them.

Focus: High Burn & Abs

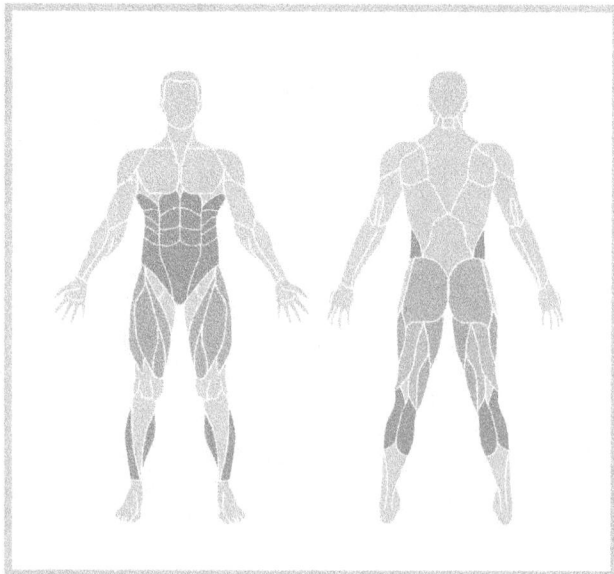

BEER BELLY

DAREBEE WORKOUT © darebee.com

LEVEL I 3 sets **LEVEL II** 5 sets **LEVEL III** 7 sets **REST** up to 2 minutes

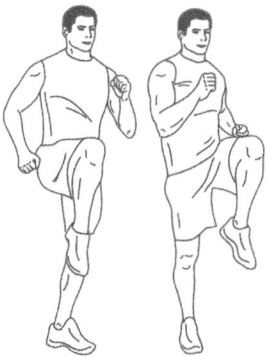

20 high knees

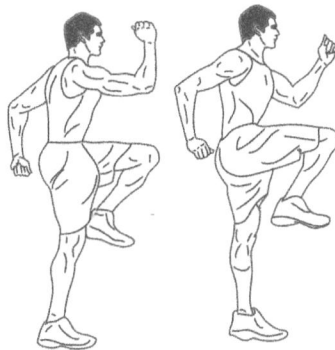

20 march steps

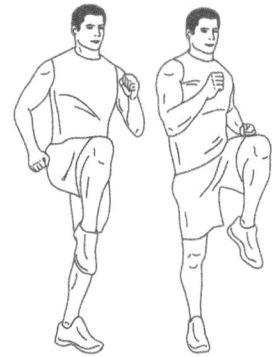

20 high knees

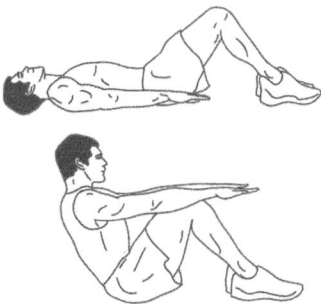

20 sit-ups

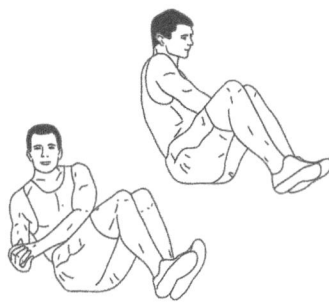

20 sitting twists

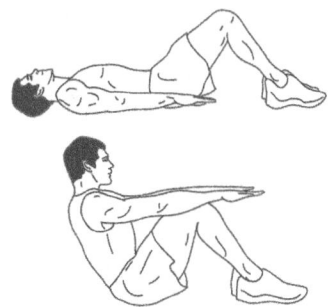

20 sit-ups

9 Bubble Butt

Glutes are powerhouses. They don't just make jeans and shorts look good, they also help athletic performance at every level. Strong glutes make you faster, stronger and capable of delivering more explosive power to virtually every movement. Bubble Butt is a workout that delivers on all these promises.

Focus: Strength & Tone

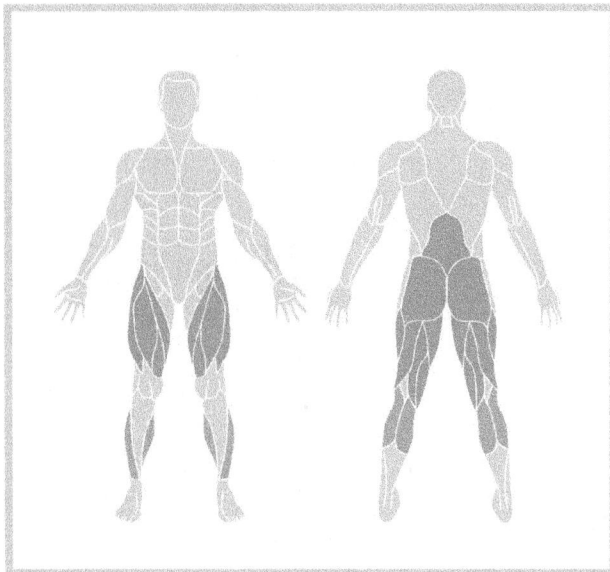

BUBBLE BUTT

DAREBEE WORKOUT
© darebee.com

2 minutes rest
between exercises

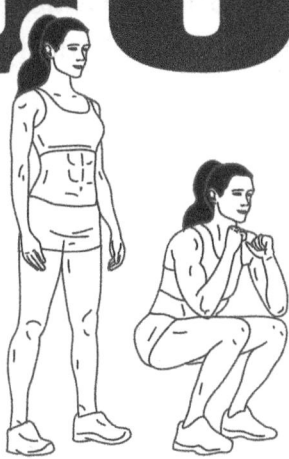

20 squats **x 4 sets** in total
20 seconds rest between sets

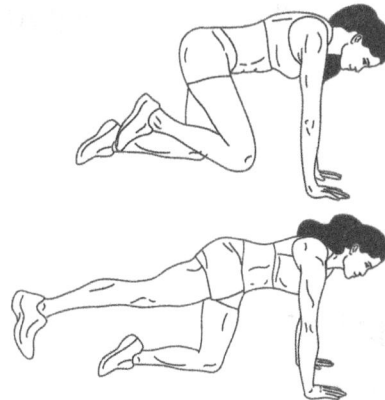

20 plank back kicks **x 4 sets** in total
2 sets per leg | 20 seconds rest

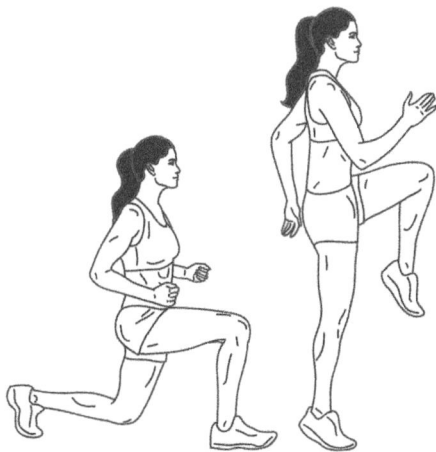

20 lunge step-ups **x 4 sets** in total
2 sets per leg | 20 seconds rest

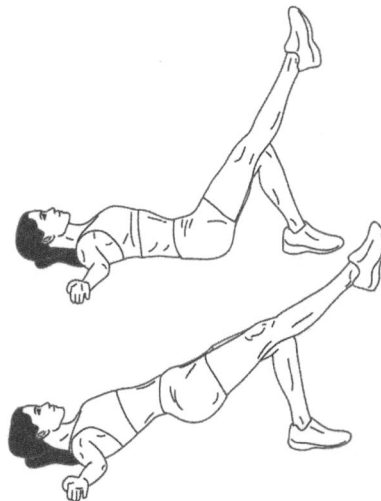

20 single leg bridges **x 4 sets** in total
2 sets per leg | 20 seconds rest

10 Burn & Build

Difficulty Level II workouts play an incredibly important role when it comes to fitness. They keep us revving when we don't really want to exercise hard. They provide great workouts for those difficult transition periods when we are beginning to level up and they help recuperation. Burn & Build does not disappoint. It does all of these things and it does them really, really well. Use it wisely and it will serve you well.

Focus: High Burn

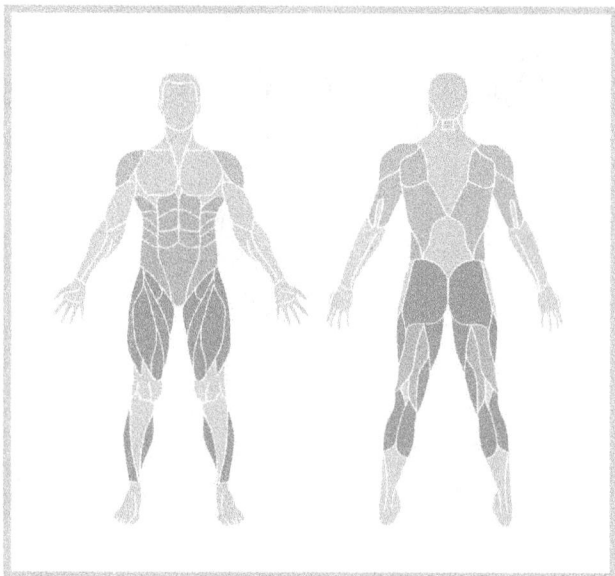

Burn & Build

DAREBEE WORKOUT © darebee.com

LEVEL I 3 sets **LEVEL II** 5 sets **LEVEL III** 7 sets **REST** up to 2 minutes

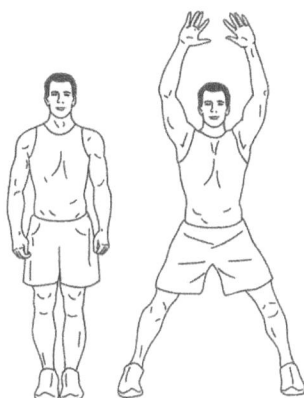

20 jumping jacks

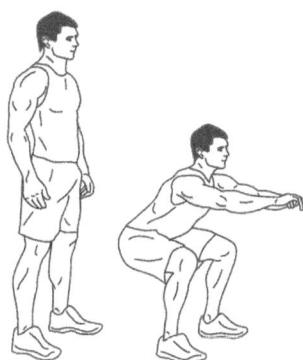

10 squats

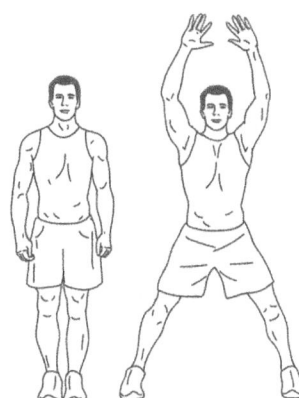

20 jumping jacks

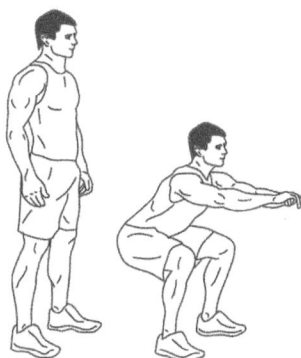

10 squats

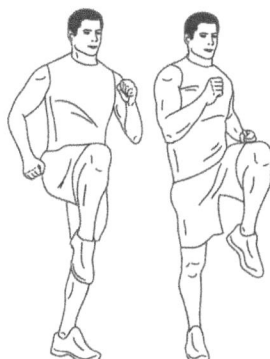

20 high knees

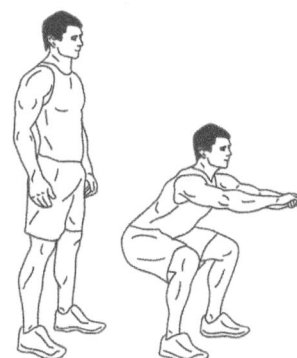

10 squats

Busy Bee

When it comes to being busy none of us has a lot of time which is why it is so important to train smart as well as hard. The Busy Bee workout makes sure you get everything you need in an intensive burst of activity that moves the entire body, challenging almost every muscle.

Focus: High Burn

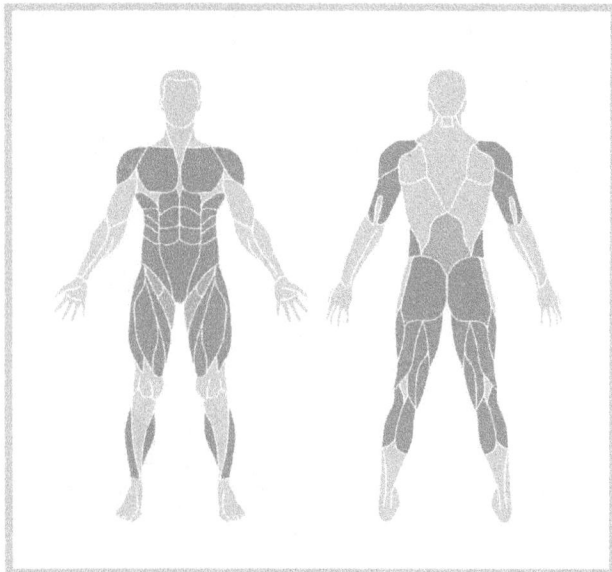

Busy Bee

DAREBEE WORKOUT © darebee.com

LEVEL I 3 sets **LEVEL II** 5 sets **LEVEL III** 7 sets **REST** up to 2 minutes

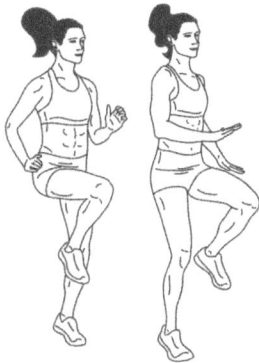

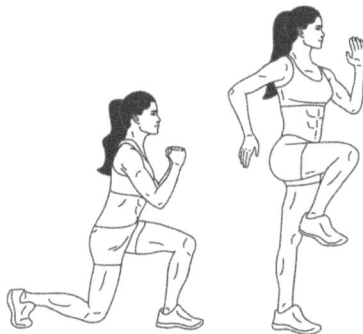

20 high knees   **10** lunge step-ups   **5** burpees

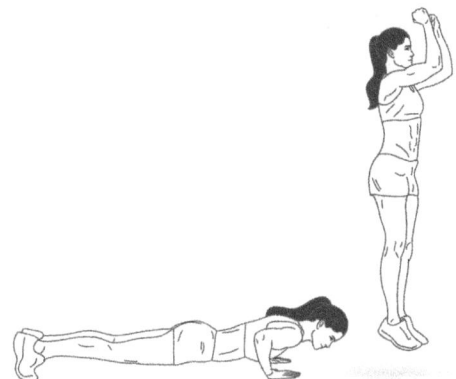

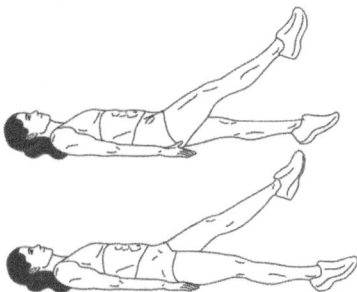

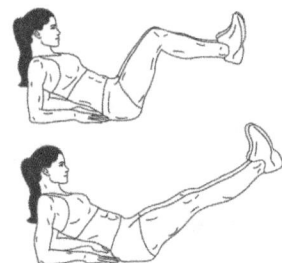

20 flutter kicks   **10** sit-ups   **5** crunch kicks

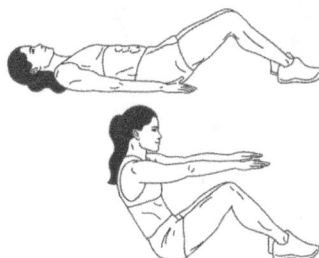

12 Cardio & Core Burn

Focus on fat burning and chisel your core with the Cardio & Core Burn Workout. You will get sweaty without ever leaving the comfort of your own home. Go as fast as you can through the circuit until the finish line, the plank. Hold the plank for as long as you possibly can - a minimum of 20 seconds.

Focus: High Burn

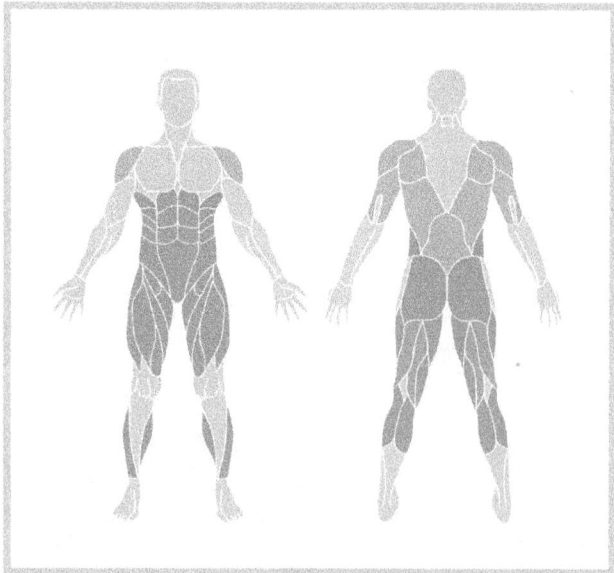

cardio
& core
burn

DAREBEE
WORKOUT
© darebee.com

Level I   3 sets
Level II   5 sets
Level III 7 sets
2 minutes rest between sets

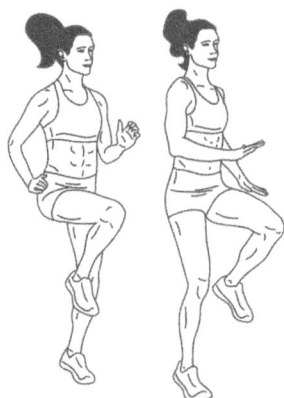

20 high knees

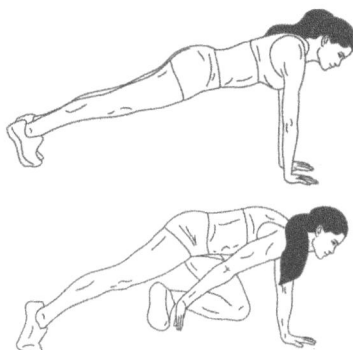

4 climber taps

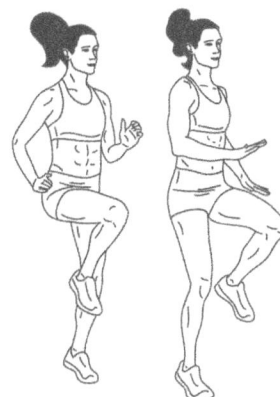

20 high knees

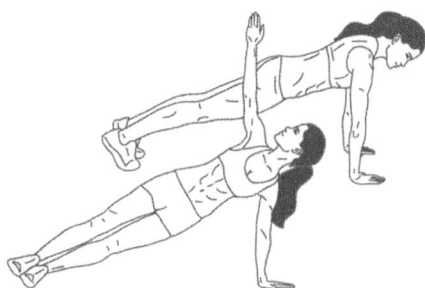

4 plank rotations

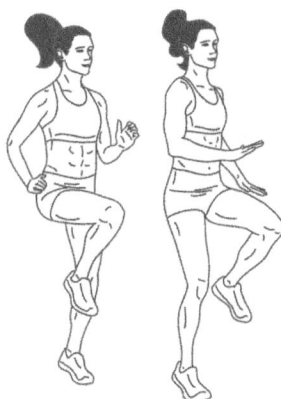

20 high knees

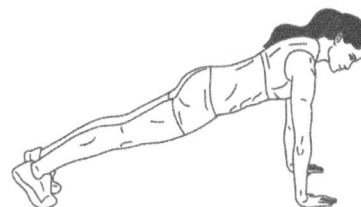

20-count plank hold

13 Cardio Fix

Cardio Fix workout is perfect for when your are short on time, recovering from an injury (or a hard workout) or just getting into circuit training cardio routines. It's perfect for beginners. Get your heart rate up, your blood flowing and sweat pouring with the Cardio Fix Workout! Keep moving until the circuit is done, don't take any breaks between exercises - go through the circuit as fast as you can for maximum results.

Focus: High Burn

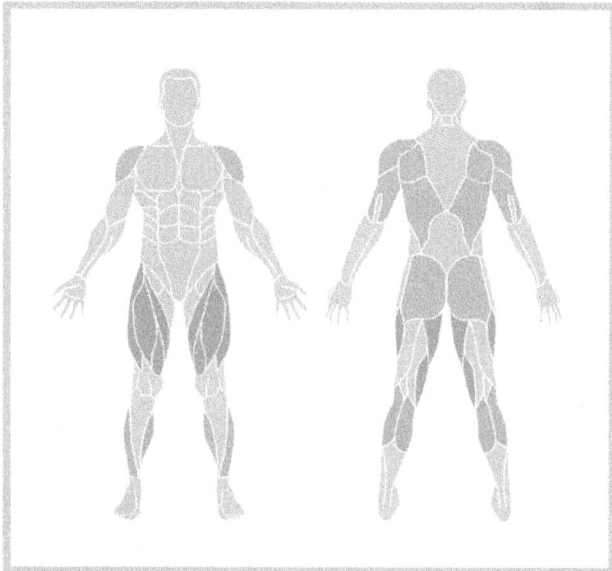

Cardio Fix

DAREBEE WORKOUT © darebee.com

LEVEL I 3 sets **LEVEL II** 5 sets **LEVEL III** 7 sets **REST** up to 2 minutes

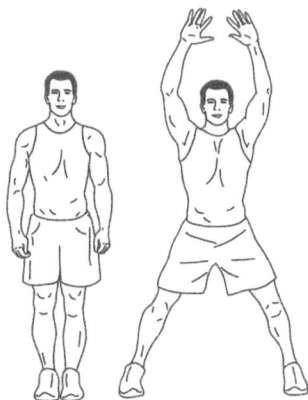

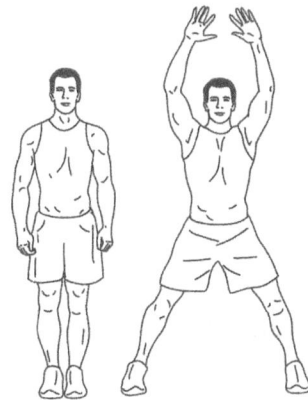

20 jumping jacks

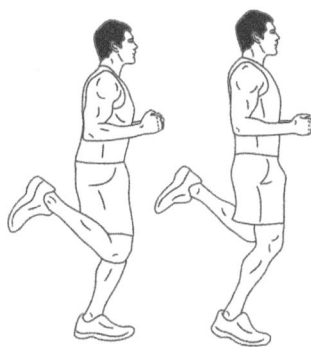

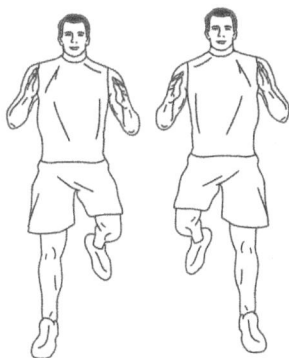

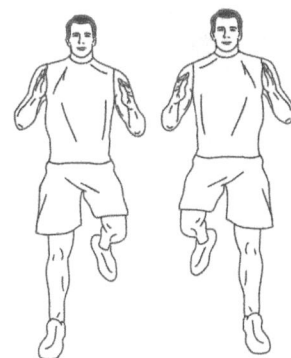

10 butt kicks

20 jumping jacks

10 side-to-side hops

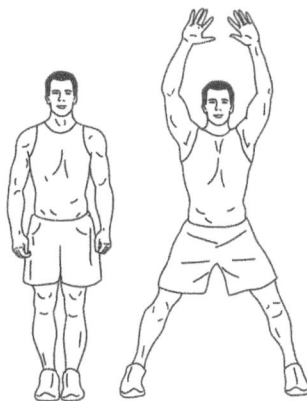

20 jumping jacks

10 side-to-side hops

14 Chopper

If someone urges you to get to the chopper you know it ain't going to be easy. For a start just calling it "chopper" means you're in a tight spot with time running out and the hordes bearing down upon you. Plus you're probably out of ammo and have nowhere to hide either. Good thing the Get To The Chopper workout is here to help you get fit enough to make it before they get you.

Focus: High Burn

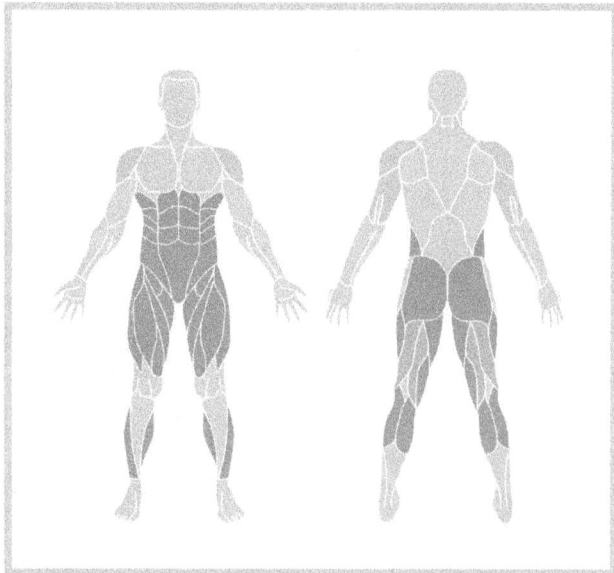

get to the chopper

DAREBEE HIIT WORKOUT © darebee.com

Level I 3 sets **Level II** 5 sets **Level III** 7 sets | 2 minutes rest

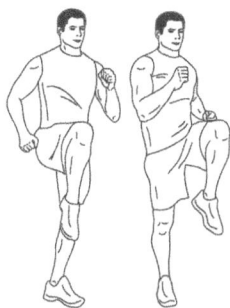

20sec high knees

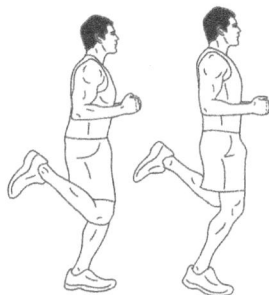

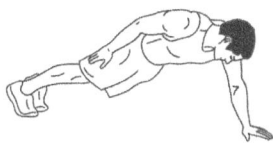

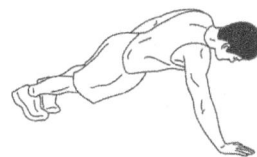

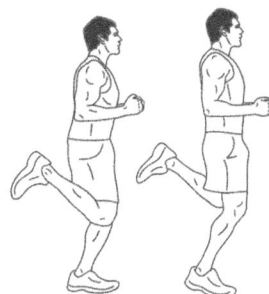

20sec butt kicks

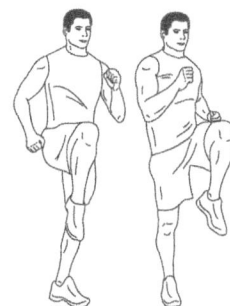

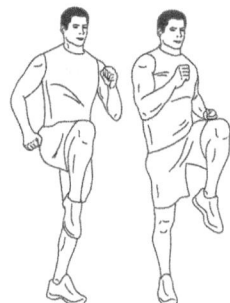

20sec high knees

20sec one-arm plank

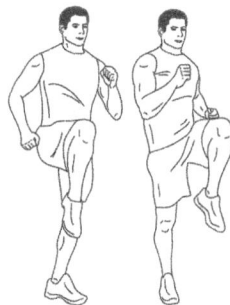

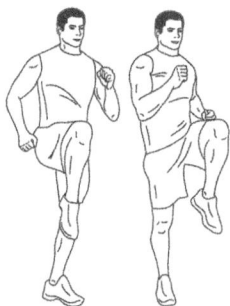

20sec high knees

20sec one-arm plank

20sec high knees

20sec butt kicks

20sec high knees

15 Coda

Take your cardio to the next level with the CODA workout. It has the best of everything and it has the worst of everything - catch your breath and dare it again! Who Dares, Wins.

Focus: High Burn

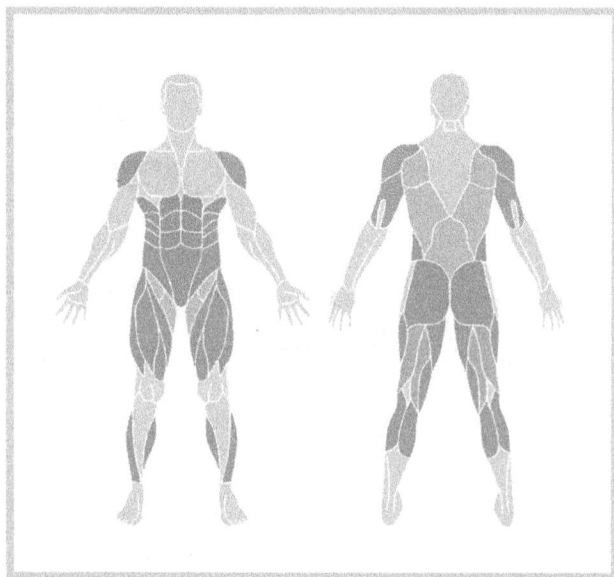

CODA

DAREBEE HIIT WORKOUT © darebee.com

Level I 3 sets **Level II** 5 sets **Level III** 7 sets | 2 minutes rest

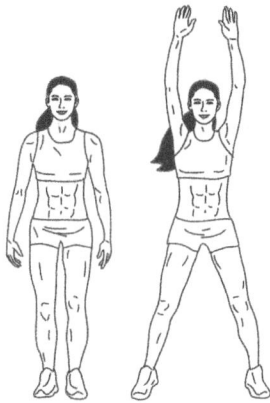

20sec jumping jacks   **20sec** plank hold   **20sec** jumping jacks

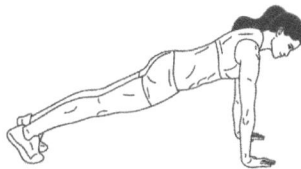

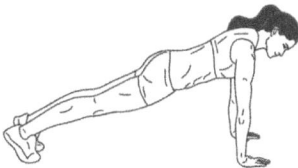

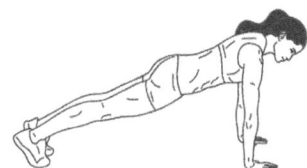

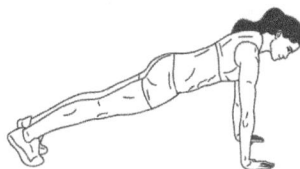

20sec plank hold   **20sec** basic burpees   **20sec** plank hold

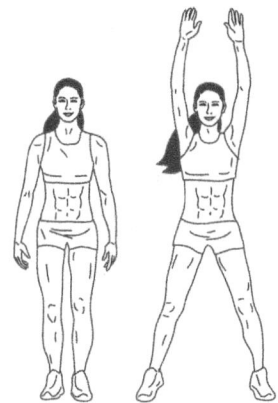

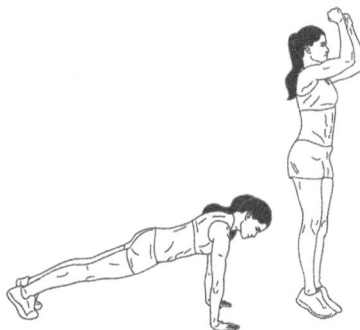

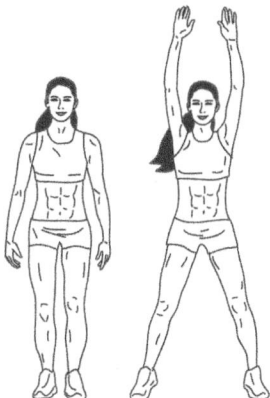

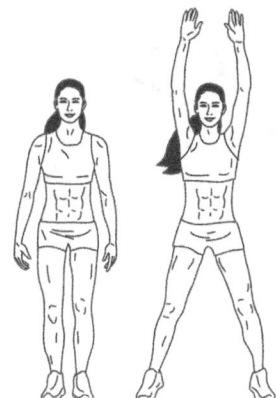

20sec jumping jacks   **20sec** plank hold   **20sec** jumping jacks

16 Combat HIIT Express

Side kicks and straight punches are the body's go-to weapons of mass destruction. They're also a great way to harness physical power, build coordination, improve balance and generate greater strength and speed. Combat HIIT Express, as the name suggests, takes you through basic punching and kicking routines at high intensity. It will make you fitter, stronger and more efficient in the way you move.

Focus: High Burn

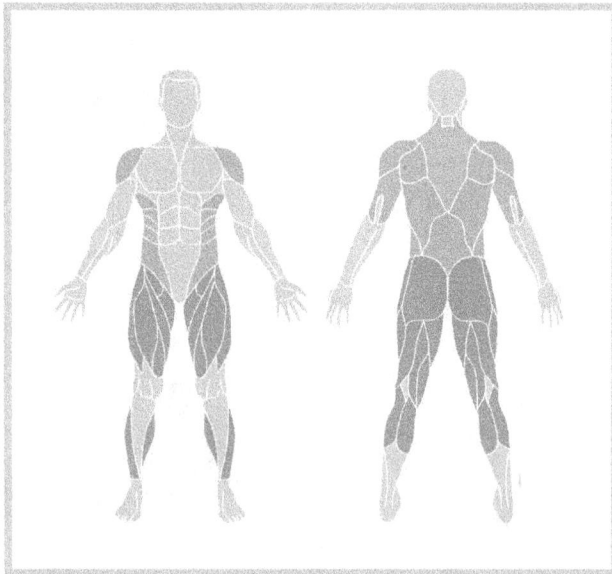

COMBAT HIIT EXPRESS

WORKOUT BY
DAREBEE
© darebee.com

Level I 3 sets
Level II 5 sets
Level III 7 sets
2 minutes rest

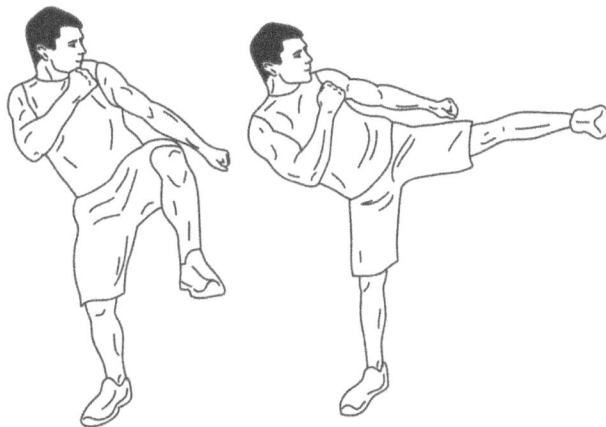

30sec side kicks

30sec punches

30sec side kicks

30sec punches

30sec side kicks

30sec punches

done

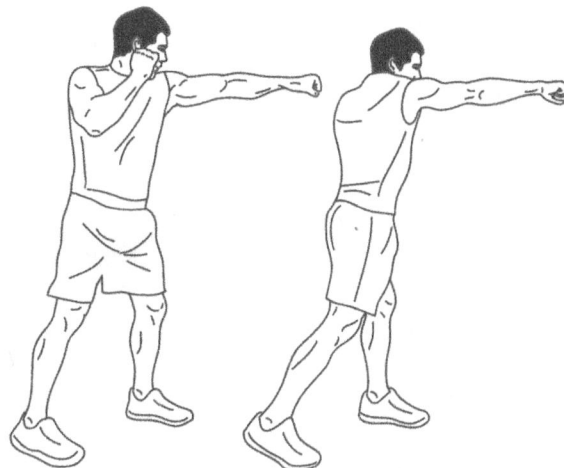

17 Core Twister

Abs need work. They require different exercises that place a different load on each of the four abdominal muscle groups. Core Twister lives up to its name. It works the core. It will push your abs. It will make you functionally more powerful by allowing the power transfer from the lower body tot he upper one and vice versa to happen with as little loss of energy as possible. To do all that, you need to do the Core Twister workout.

Focus: Abs & Core

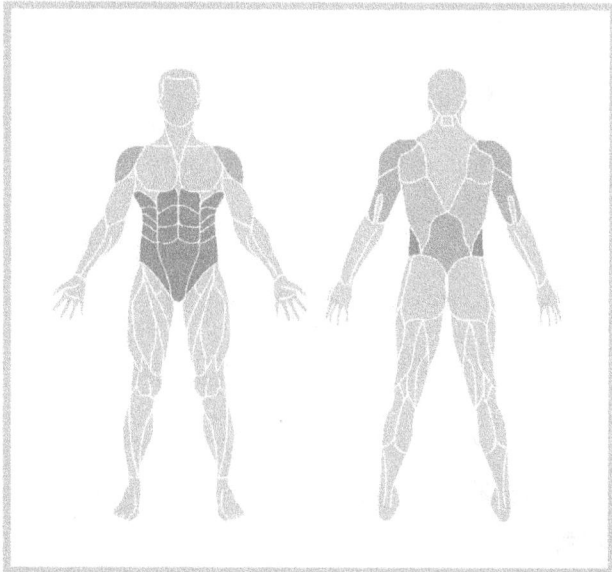

CORE TWISTER

DAREBEE WORKOUT © darebee.com

Switch sides and repeat the sequence again.

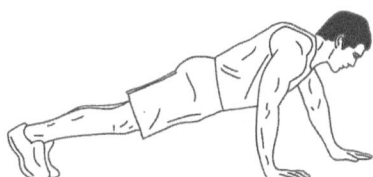

20 seconds
staggered plank hold

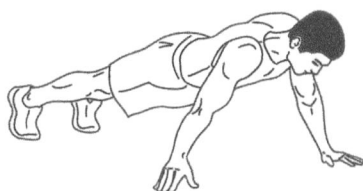

20 seconds
archer plank hold

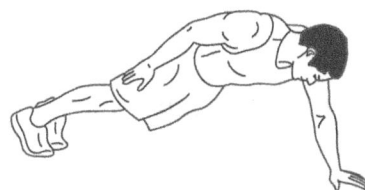

20 seconds
one-arm plank hold

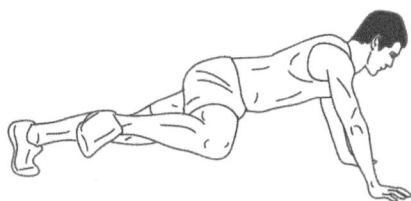

20 seconds
knee-to-the-side
plank hold

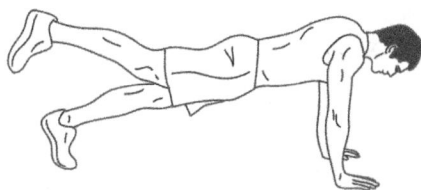

20 seconds
raised leg plank hold

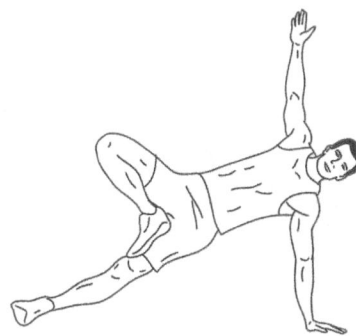

20 seconds
tucked-in
side plank hold

Critical Hit

When put together in the right combo that loads muscle groups and taxes the aerobic system combat skills are the fastest way there is to achieve gains in speed, balance, coordination and power. Critical Hit does not disappoint. It loads the body's major muscle groups, taxes VO2 capacity and tests endurance and recovery time. Put this one on your horizon and work at it until you can do it with a smile all the way.

Focus: Combat

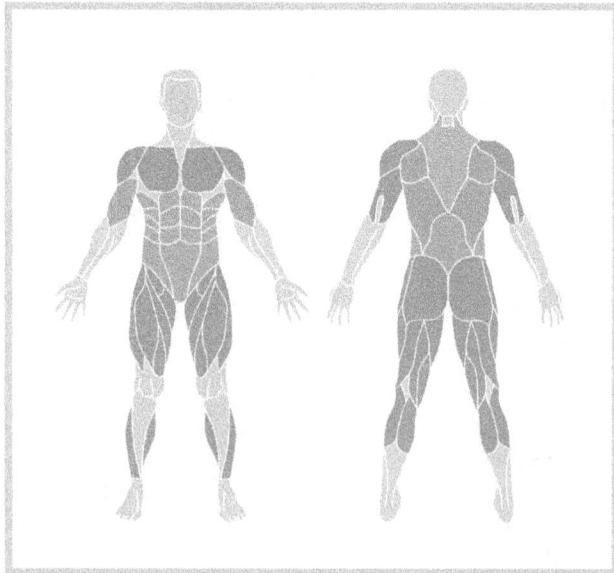

CRITICAL HIT

DAREBEE WORKOUT © darebee.com

LEVEL I 3 sets **LEVEL II** 5 sets **LEVEL III** 7 sets **REST** up to 2 minutes

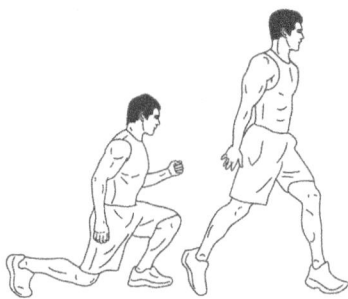

10 jumping lunges

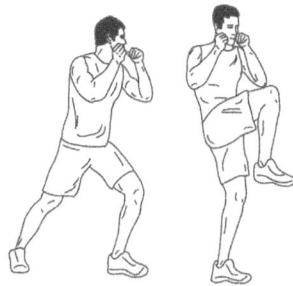

20 knee strikes

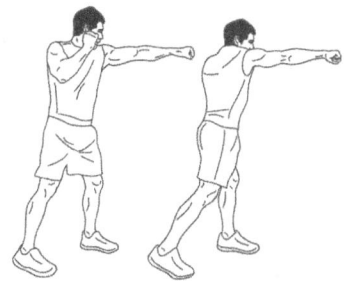

20 punches

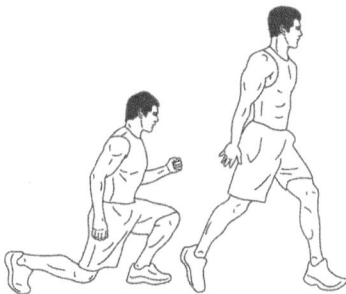

10 jumping lunges

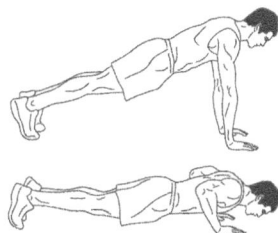

20 push-ups

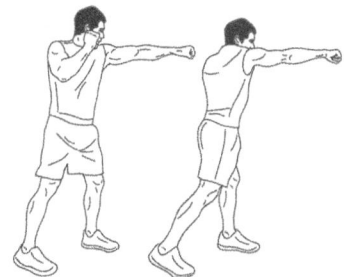

20 punches

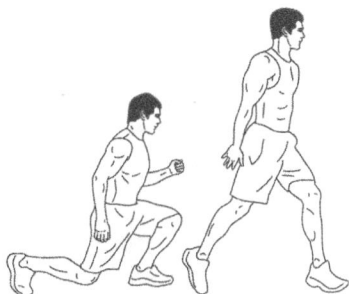

10 jumping lunges

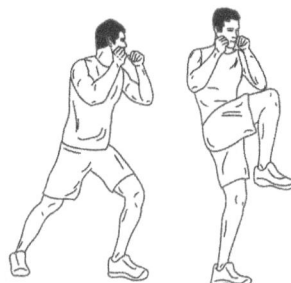

20 knee strikes

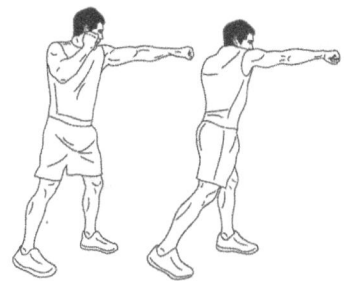

20 punches

19   Crushing It!

Crushing It! is a fun yet grueling combat workout. It's simple yet it recruits all major muscle groups. It demands concentration and a decent amount of coordination. Simple moves + decent numbers + smart circuit = excellent ROI. Mind your form and go slow when doing push-ups. You don't want speed here, you want to focus on your technique and harness gravity to help you hyperload and challenge your muscles.

Focus: Combat

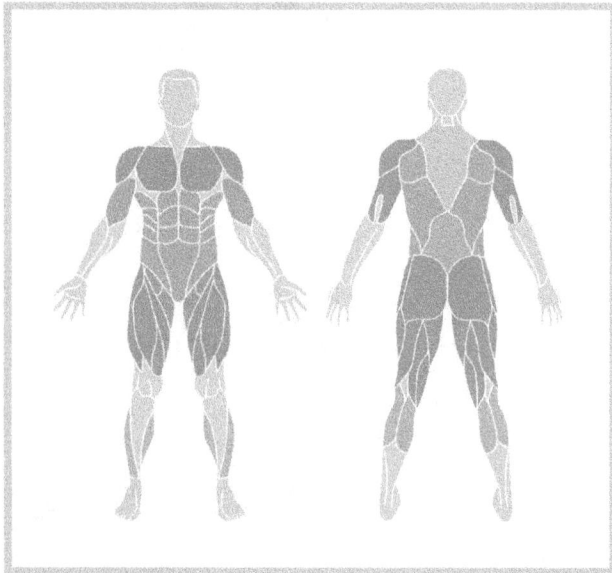

Crushing it!

DAREBEE WORKOUT © darebee.com

LEVEL I 3 sets **LEVEL II** 5 sets **LEVEL III** 7 sets **REST** up to 2 minutes

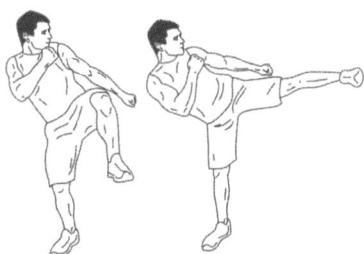

10 side kicks (left)

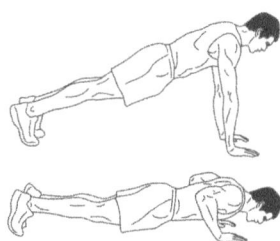

10 push-ups

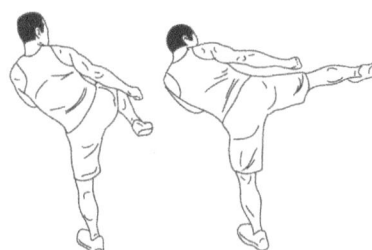

10 side kicks (right)

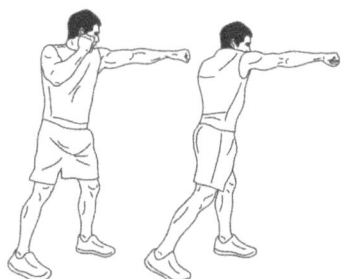

20 punches

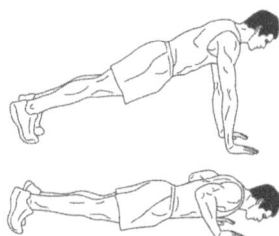

10 push-ups

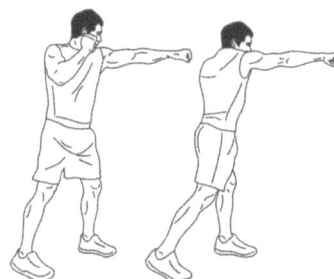

20 punches

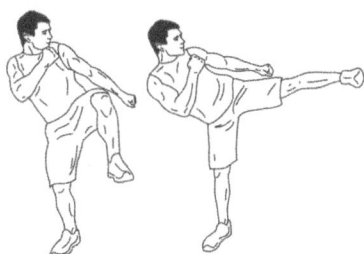

10 side kicks (left)

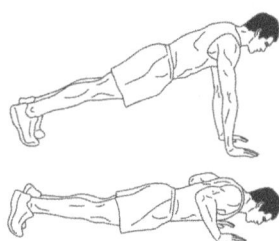

10 push-ups

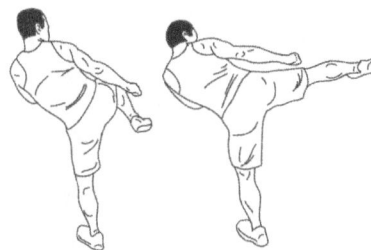

10 side kicks (right)

Cyberpunk

Sensibilities of control, focus, self-determination and transformation spill over into real life. The Cyberpunk workout is here to help you realize them all.

Focus: Strength & Tone

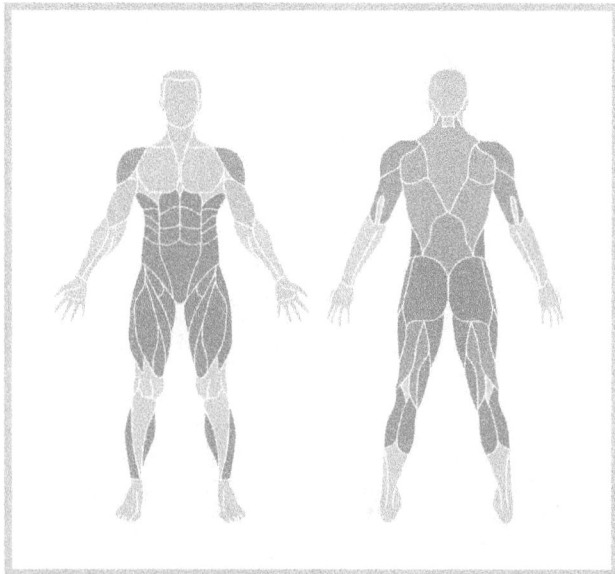

CYBERPUNK

DAREBEE WORKOUT © darebee.com

LEVEL I 3 sets **LEVEL II** 5 sets **LEVEL III** 7 sets **REST** up to 2 minutes

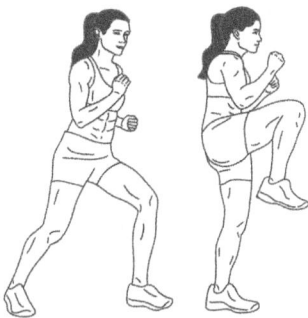

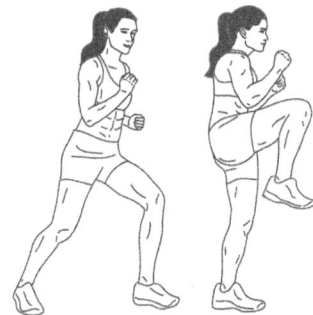

20 knee strikes

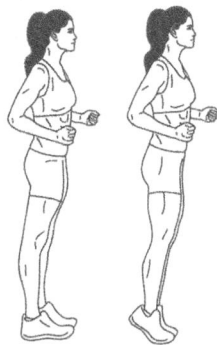

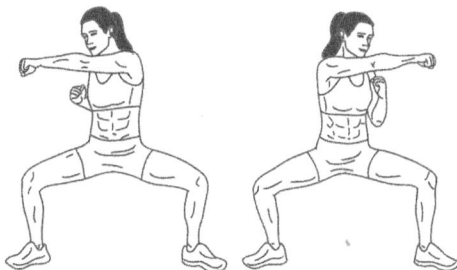

6 calf raises

20 knee strikes

20 squat hold punches

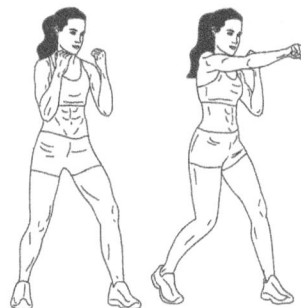

20 punches

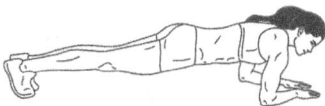

10 elbow plank step outs

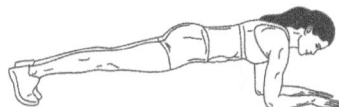

6 elbow plank knee-ins

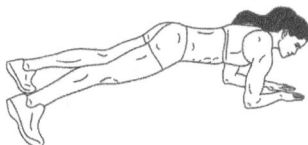

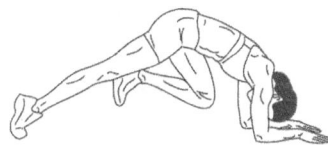

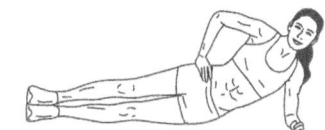

10 side bridges

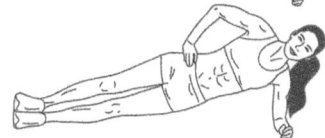

21   Deathsquad

Deathsquad is a full body, strength workout that begins to exert its influence on the body's muscles shortly after you get through the very first set. Although it's just level III in difficulty, it doesn't take long before fatigue kicks in and then you're working through that figurative wall the other side of which lies the physical strength you crave.

Focus: Strength & Tone

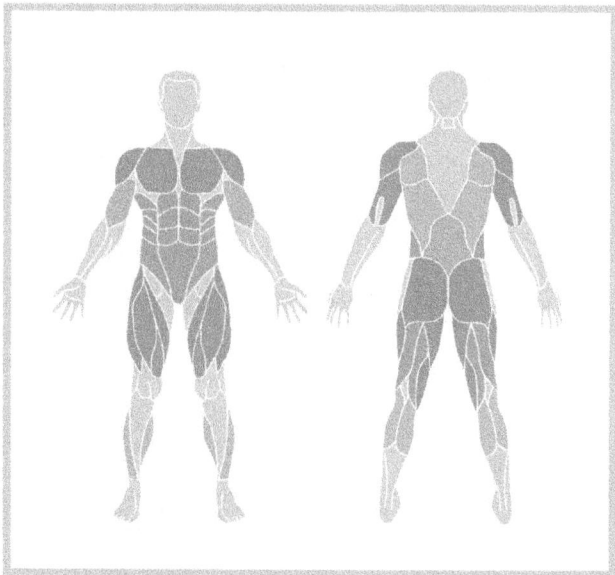

DEATHSQUAD

DAREBEE WORKOUT © darebee.com

LEVEL I 3 sets **LEVEL II** 5 sets **LEVEL III** 7 sets **REST** up to 2 minutes

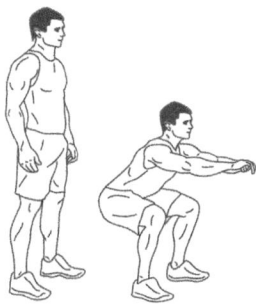

15 squats

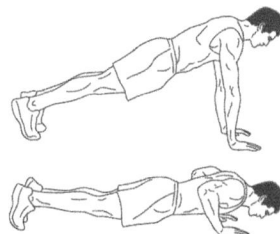

5 push-ups

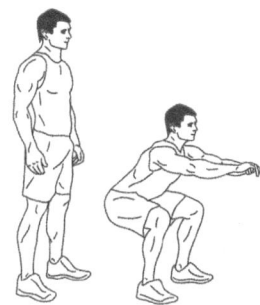

15 squats

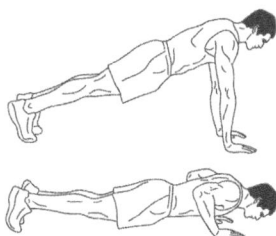

5 push-ups

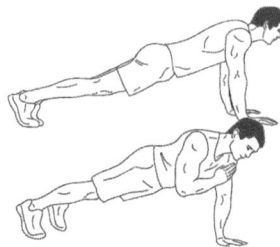

30 shoulder taps

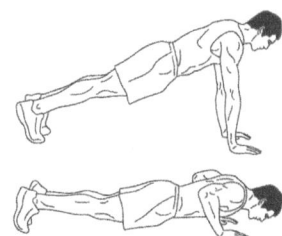

5 push-ups

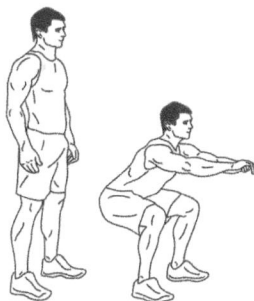

15 squats

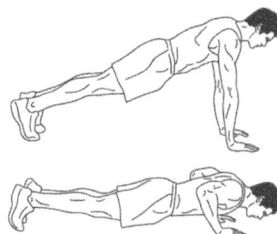

5 push-ups

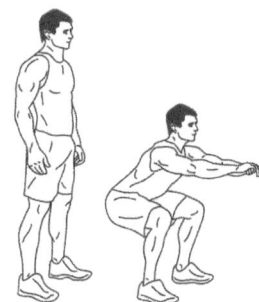

15 squats

22 Defiant

Reach for the stars! Be defiant and keep on moving forward until you reach your goals. Make sure you lower your knee all the way to the floor, almost touching it, when performing lunges. Go slow throughout the circuit and mind your form.

Focus: Strength & Tone

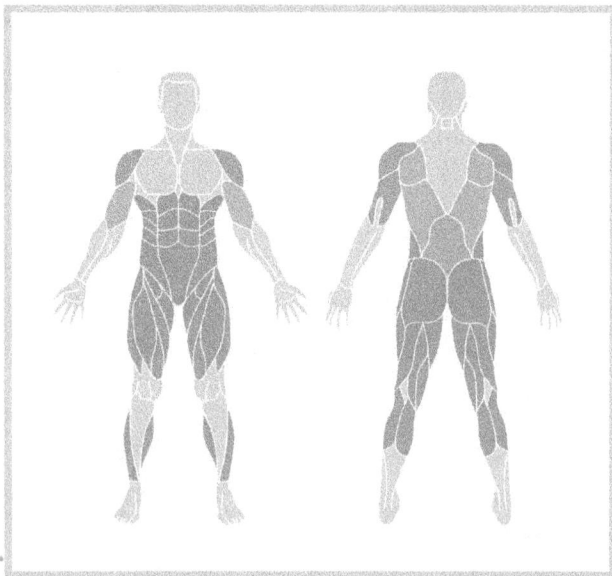

DEFIANT

DAREBEE WORKOUT © darebee.com

LEVEL I 3 sets **LEVEL II** 5 sets **LEVEL III** 7 sets **REST** up to 2 minutes

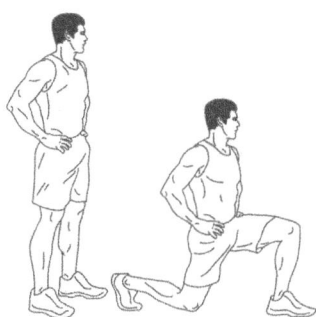

10 lunges

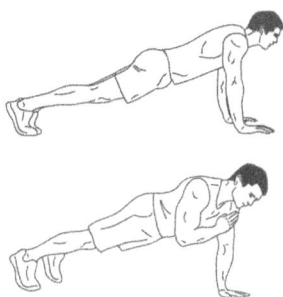

10 shoulder taps

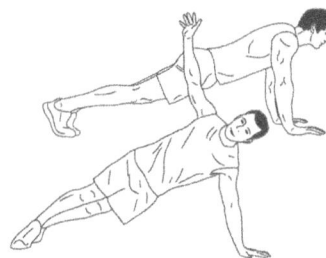

10 plank rotations

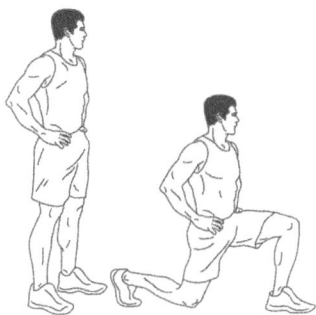

10 lunges

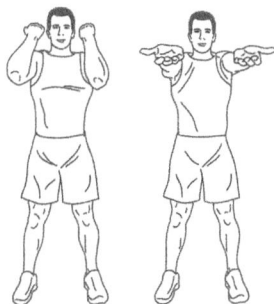

30 bicep extensions

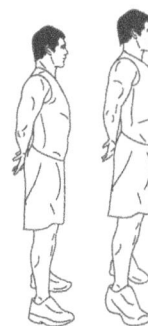

10 calf raises

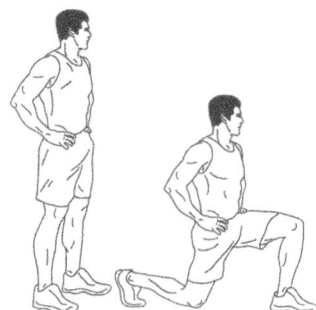

10 lunges

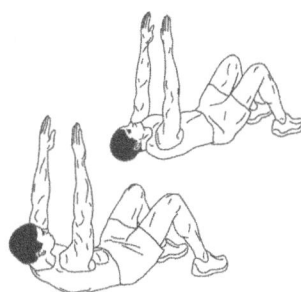

10 high crunches

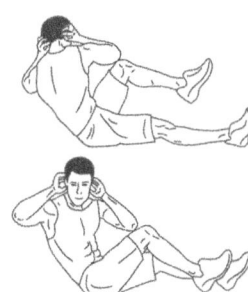

10 knee-to-elbows

23 Do Over

A difficulty level II workout can still deliver solid physical performance benefits, even to advanced fitness athletes if it is performed at Level III with EC and that's because, like each workout it challenges the body differently forcing a new adaptation response which means it helps you get fitter regardless. Plus this is a workout which can be performed by anyone at virtually any level of fitness which means it is also a good challenge to have on your horizon.

Focus: High Burn

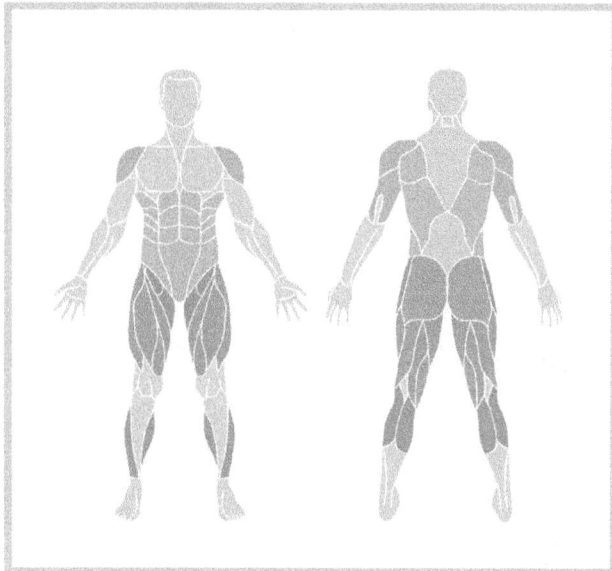

THE DO OVER

DAREBEE WORKOUT © darebee.com

LEVEL I 3 sets **LEVEL II** 5 sets **LEVEL III** 7 sets **REST** up to 2 minutes

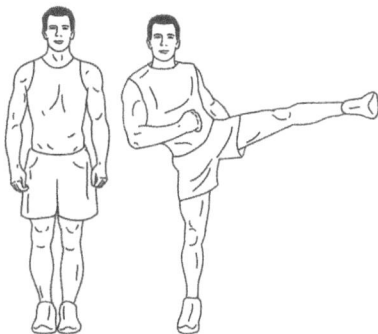

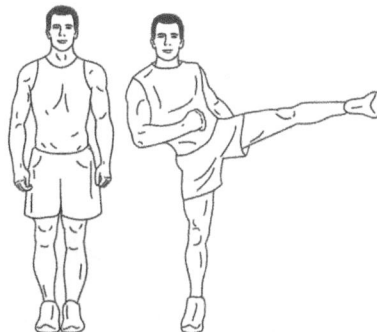

20 side leg raises

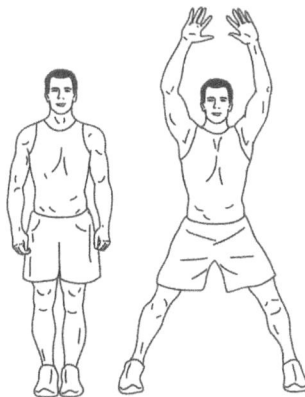

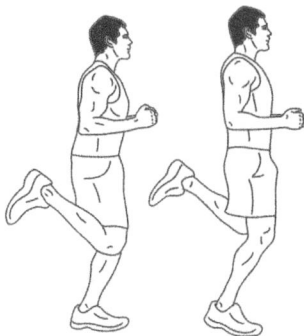

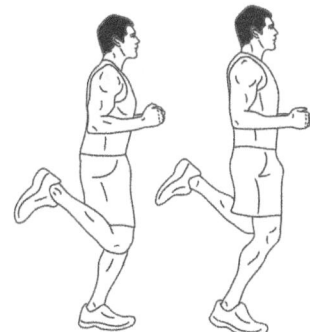

20 jumping jacks

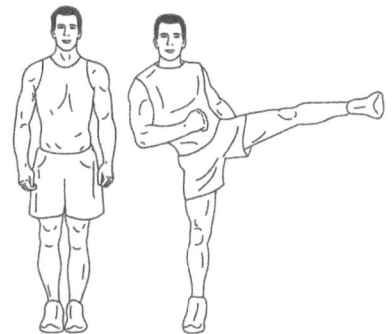

20 side leg raises

20 butt kicks

20 side leg raises

20 butt kicks

24 Expedited Delivery

Expedited delivery is zippy and even the floor exercises are designed to put a load on muscles ans tendons that are used in the rest of the workout. That makes it a challenge to get through without a groan 9or two) which means it will work to bring up your body temperature and put you in the sweatzone, fast.

Focus: High Burn

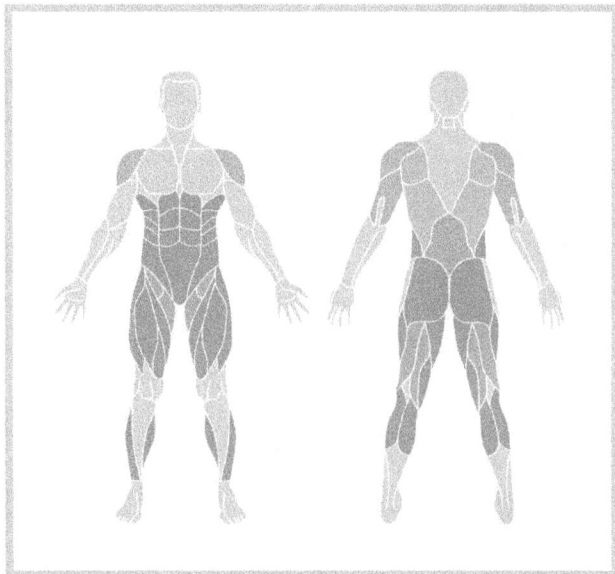

EXPEDITED DELIVERY

DAREBEE HIIT WORKOUT © darebee.com

Level I 3 sets **Level II** 5 sets **Level III** 7 sets | 2 minutes rest

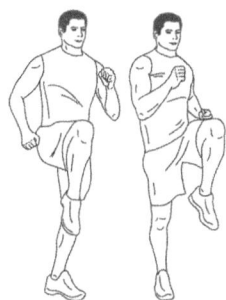

20sec high knees

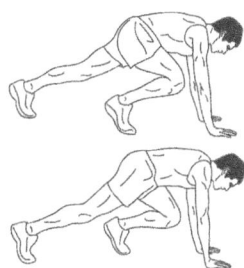

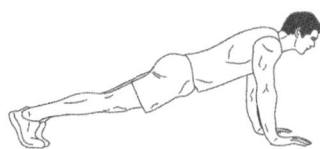

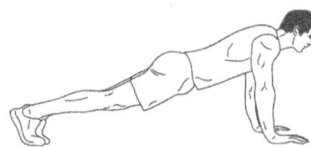

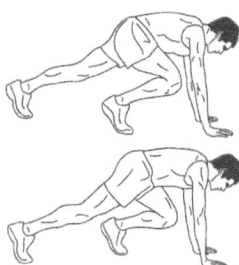

20sec climbers

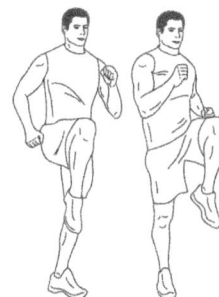

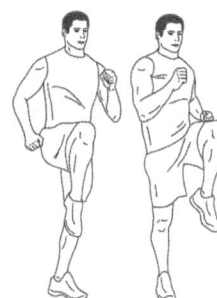

20sec high knees

20sec plank hold

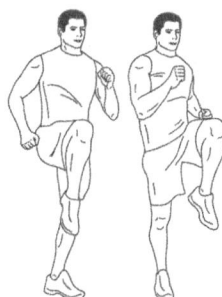

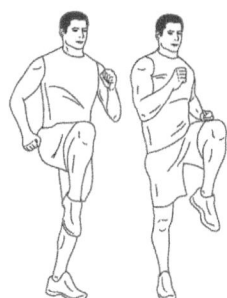

20sec high knees

20sec plank hold

20sec high knees

20sec climbers

20sec high knees

25 Extra Spice

Life is meant to be spiced up which is why Extra Spice is a total body workout that comes with the usual focus on form and quality of movement through every set.

Focus: High Burn

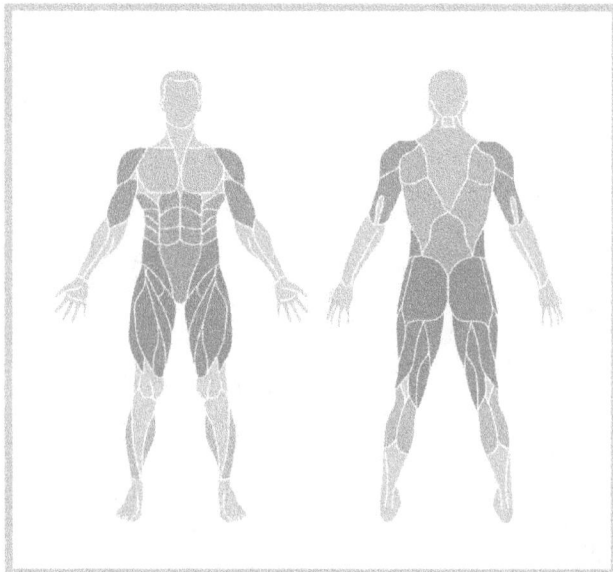

EXTRA SPICE

DAREBEE WORKOUT
© darebee.com
Level I 3 sets
Level II 5 sets
Level III 7 sets
2 minutes rest

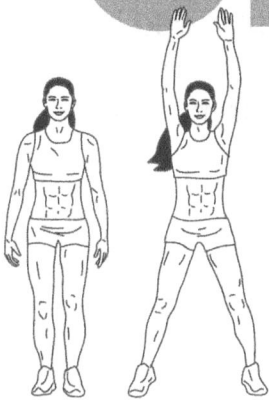

15 jumping jacks

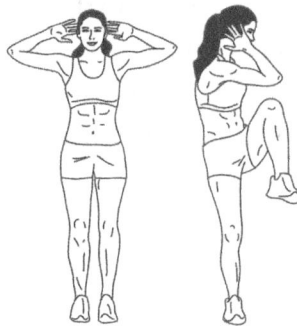

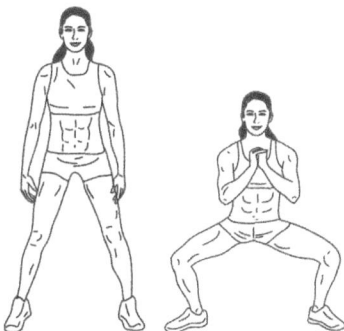

10 knee-to-elbows

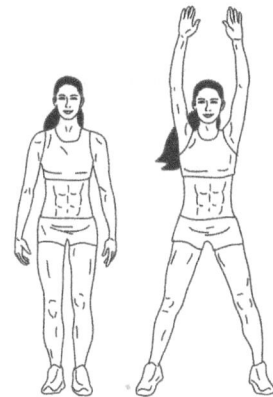

15 jumping jacks

10 goblet squats

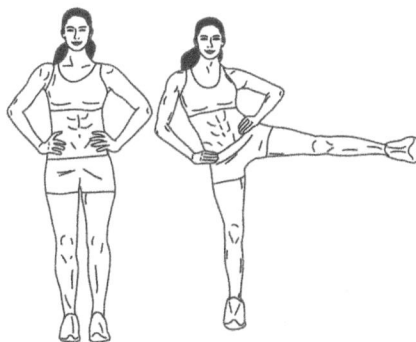

10 side leg raises

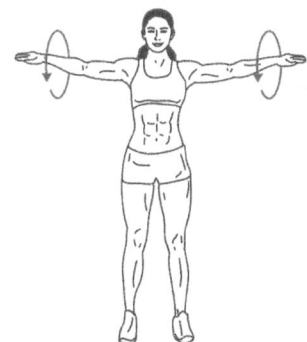

15 raised arm circles

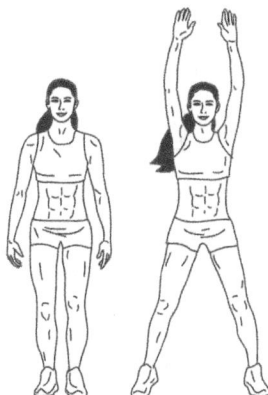

15 jumping jacks

26   Fab Abs

The abs and core are the junction at which lower body strength is translated into upper body power. But for that to happen you need strong abs and a strong core. Fab Abs works all of that in a dynamic and static fashion. The cross-mix delivers a potent abs workout that demands you raise your knees to waist height during High Knees and keep your body as absolutely straight as you possibly can during plank.

Focus: High Burn & Abs

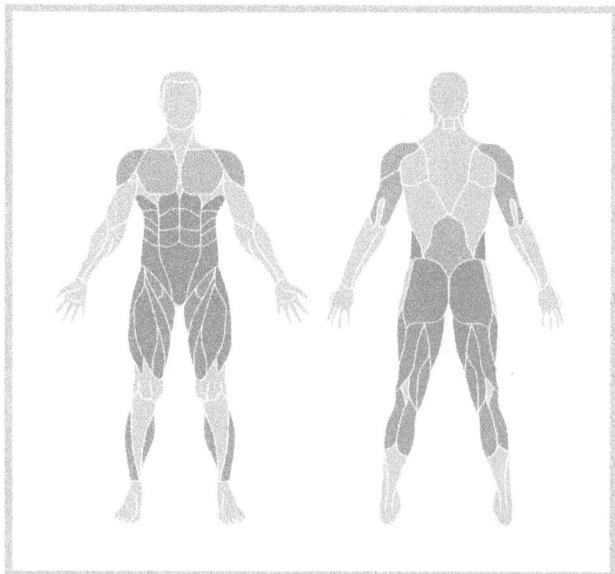

FAB ABS

DAREBEE HIIT WORKOUT © darebee.com

Level I 3 sets **Level II** 5 sets **Level III** 7 sets | 2 minutes rest

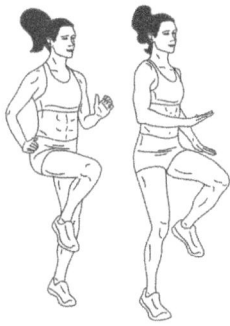

20sec high knees | **20sec** elbow plank hold | **20sec** high knees

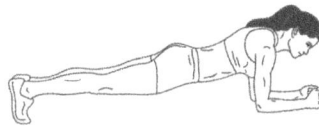

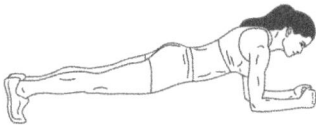

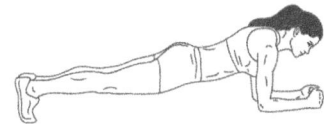

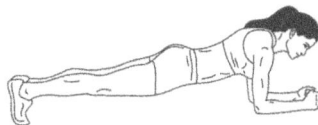

20sec elbow plank hold | **20sec** climbers | **20sec** elbow plank hold

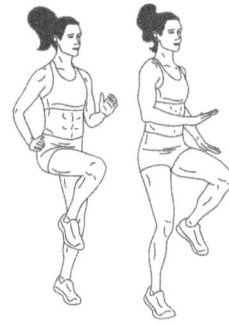

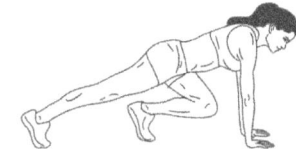

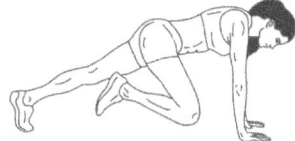

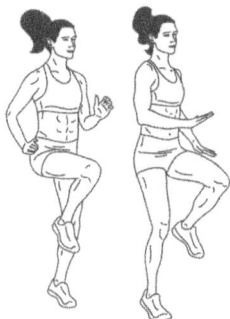

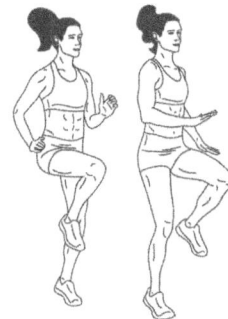

20sec high knees | **20sec** elbow plank hold | **20sec** high knees

Feel Good

Exercise is one of the best ways to get an instant mood boost. This quick and easy workout is just what doctor prescribed. Go flat out throughout the circuit, it's going to be worth it!

Focus: High Burn

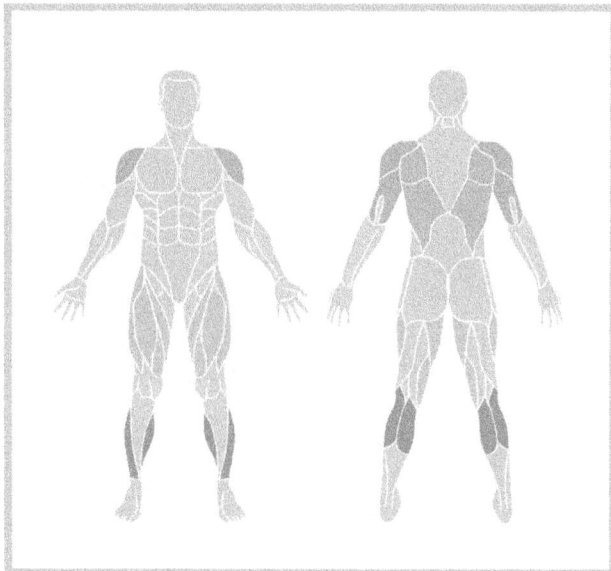

feelgood

DAREBEE WORKOUT © darebee.com

LEVEL I 3 sets **LEVEL II** 4 sets **LEVEL III** 5 sets **REST** up to 2 minutes

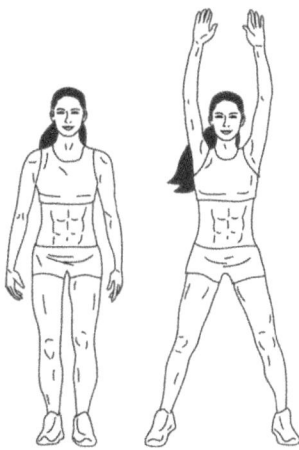

10 jumping jacks

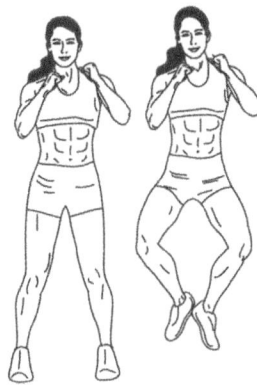

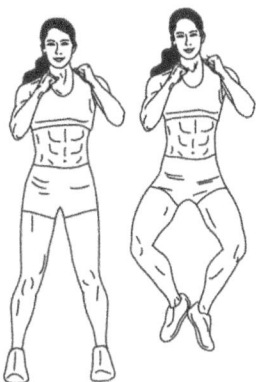

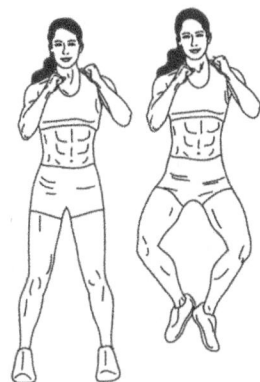

2 hop heel clicks

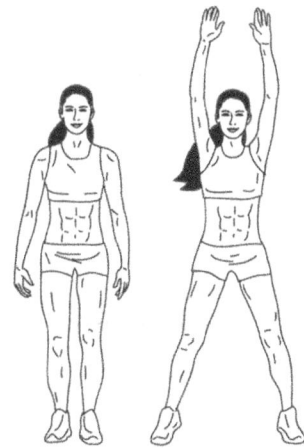

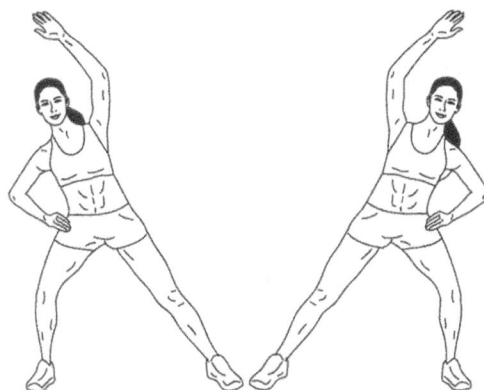

10 jumping jacks

2 hop heel clicks

10 side jacks

2 hop heel clicks

28 Femme Fatale

Get into character, be a special agent and feel empowered, capable and dangerous with the Femme Fatale workout. Combat moves, groundwork and tendon strengthening exercises will transform your body into one focused, fit, fighting machine.

Focus: Strength & Tone

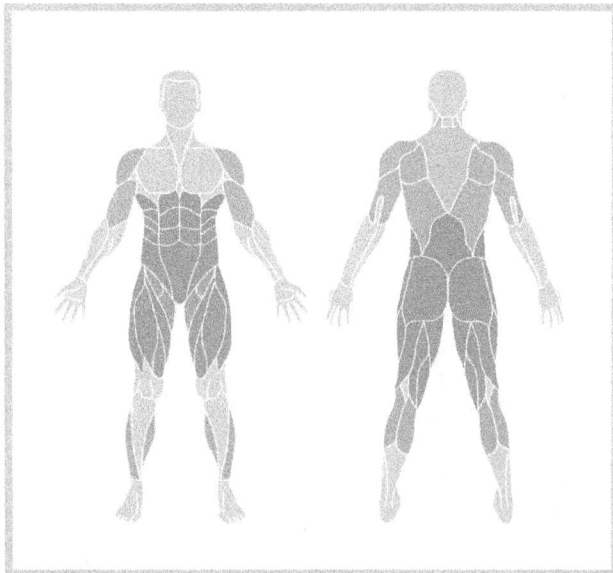

FEMME FATALE

DAREBEE
WORKOUT
© darebee.com
LEVEL I 3 sets
LEVEL II 5 sets
LEVEL III 7 sets
2 minutes rest

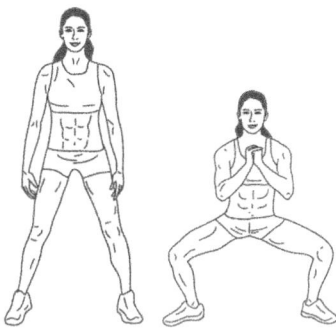

10 goblet squats

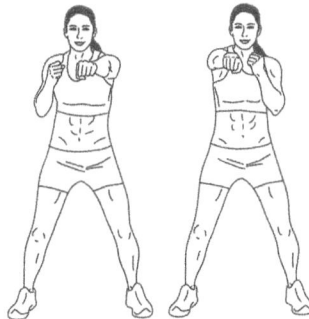

20 punches

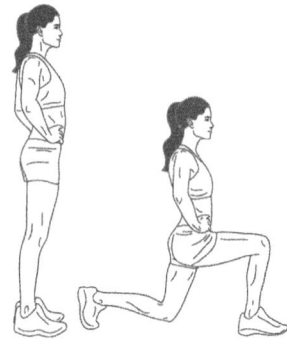

10 lunges

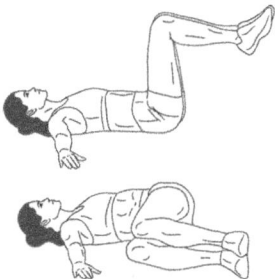

10 half wipers

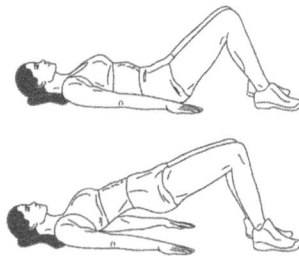

10 bridges

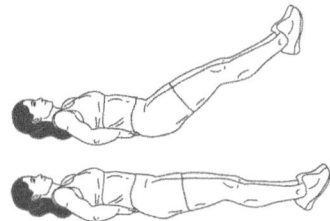

10 leg raises

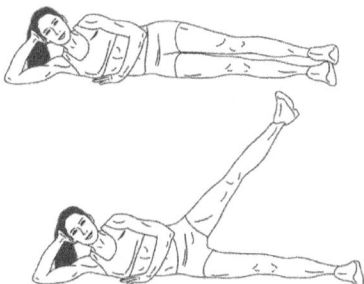

20 side leg raises

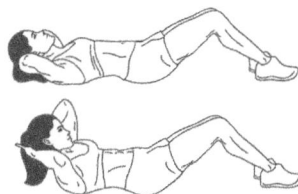

20 crunches

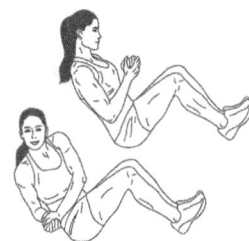

20 sitting twists

29 Fresh Start

Fresh Start is the kind of workout you should be looking at if you're getting back into training after a lay-off due to injury or other circumstances. It's light, it's fast, it's energizing and it will help your body remember how it should move.

Focus: High Burn

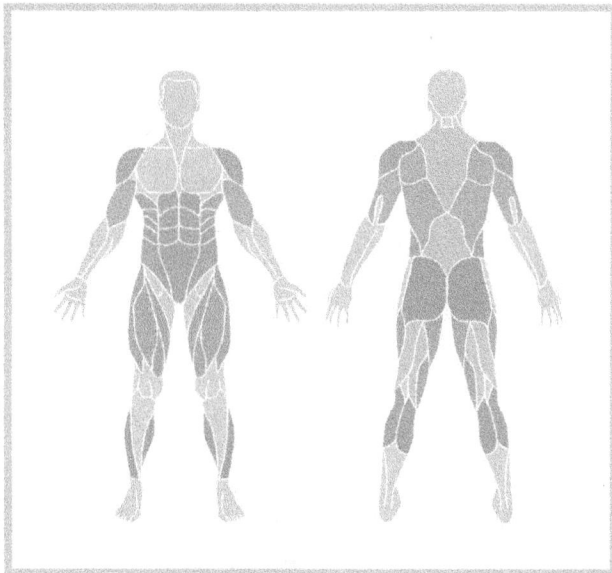

FRESH START

DAREBEE WORKOUT © darebee.com

LEVEL I 3 sets **LEVEL II** 5 sets **LEVEL III** 7 sets **REST** up to 2 minutes

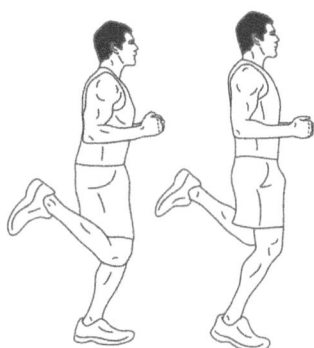

10 butt kicks

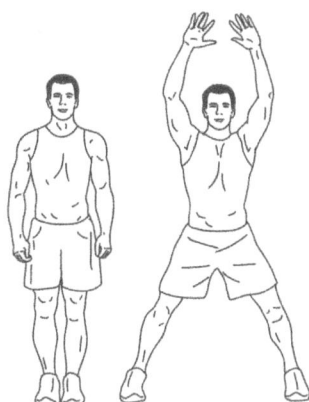

10 jumping jacks

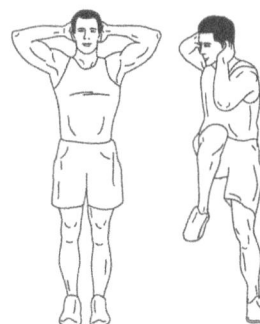

10 knee-to-elbow

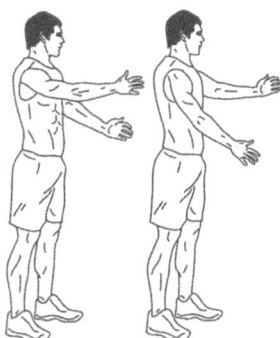

20 scissor chops

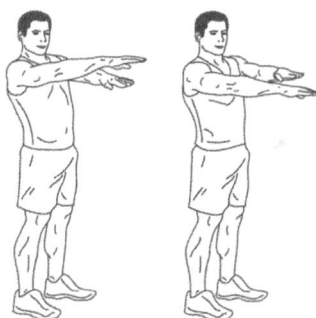

20 arm scissors

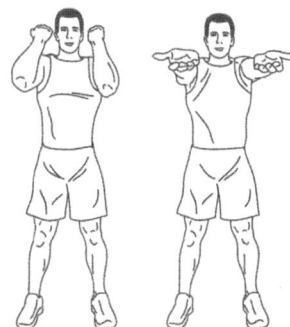

20 bicep extensions

30

Genesis

It's always hard in the beginning but if you stick with it, in the end it's all worth it. The Genesis workout is pure fire, it will break you to remake you. Bear with it, give it your all, persevere and, once you conquer it, nothing will ever feel like too much to overcome. This is how toughness is nurtured and how iron will is forged. Keep moving, as fast as you can until the time is done, catch your breath and do it again. Bring your knees up as high as you can, as far in as you can and don't forget to breathe!

Focus: High Burn

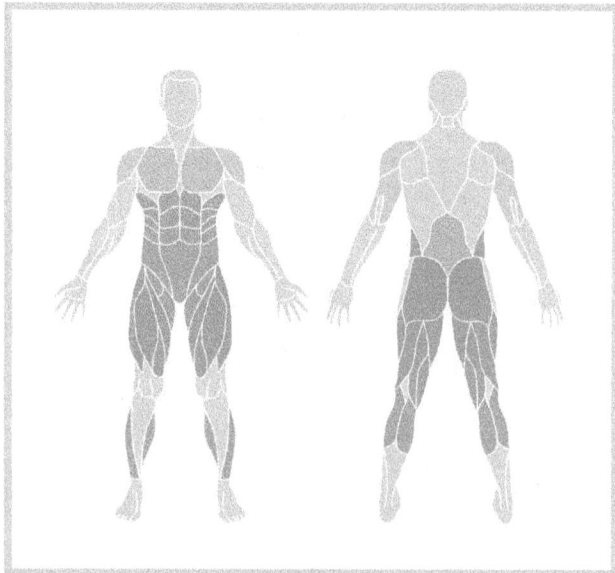

GENESIS

DAREBEE HIIT WORKOUT © darebee.com

Level I 3 sets **Level II** 5 sets **Level III** 7 sets | 2 minutes rest

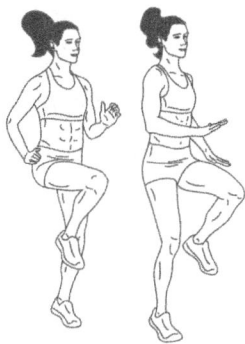

20sec high knees

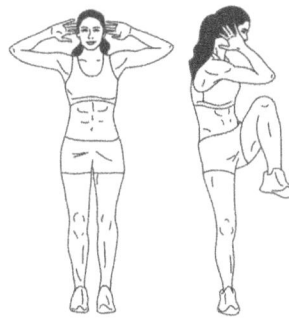

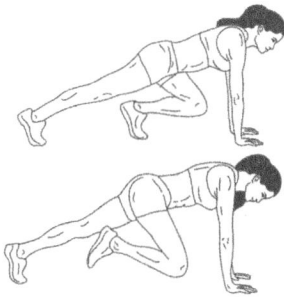

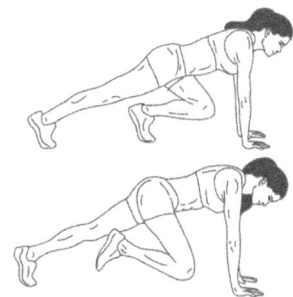

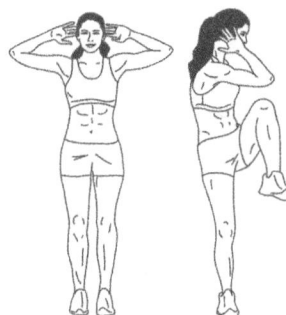

20sec knee-to-elbows

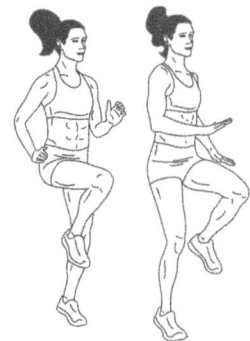

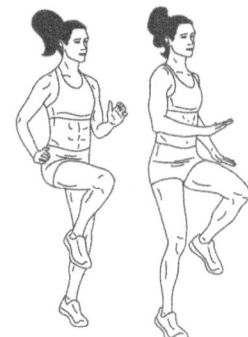

20sec high knees

20sec climbers

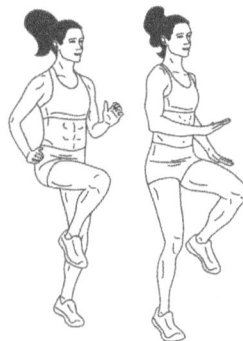

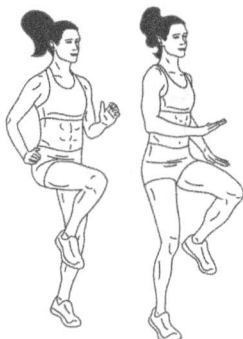

20sec high knees

20sec climbers

20sec high knees

20sec knee-to-elbows

20sec high knees

31

Get It Done

This workout is perfect for when you just need to - Get It Done. It will challenge your lungs and work your core without overtaxing your system delivering just the right amount of burn, at the right time. It's fairly easy to follow, there are no complex moves, but it will work your entire body nonetheless. Keep your arm up throughout the second row and keep your elbows pointing forward during bicep extensions - don't drop your arms down, for maximum results.

Focus: High Burn

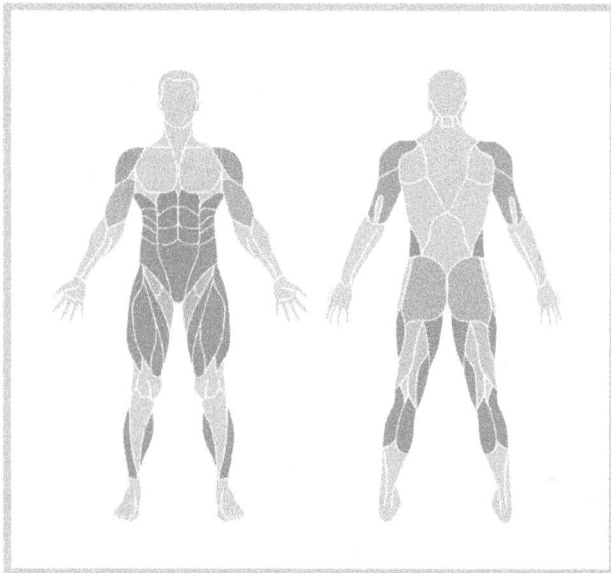

Get it done

DAREBEE HIIT WORKOUT © darebee.com

Level I 3 sets **Level II** 5 sets **Level III** 7 sets

2 minutes rest between sets

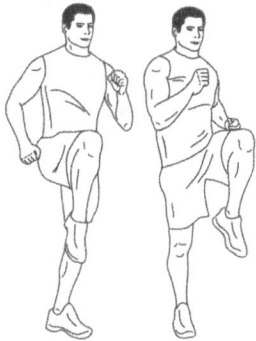

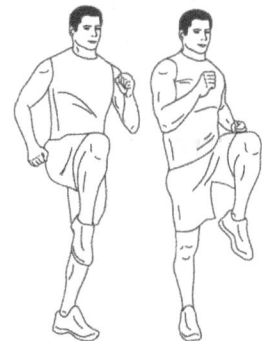

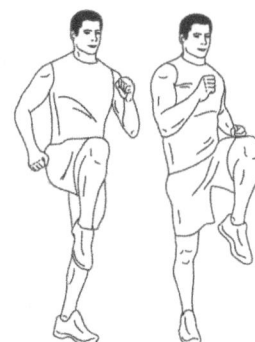

20sec high knees   **20sec** plank hold   **20sec** high knees

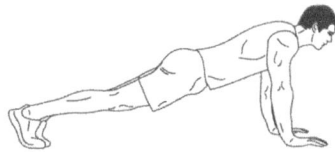

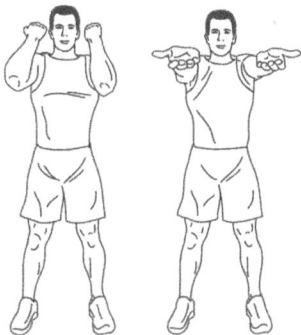

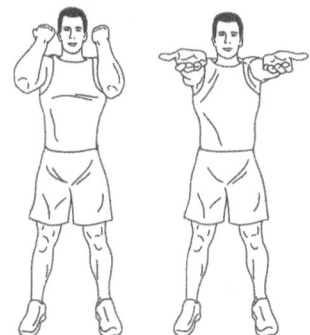

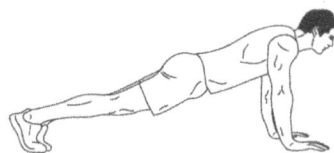

20sec bicep extensions   **20sec** raised arm hold   **20sec** bicep extensions

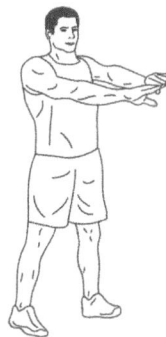

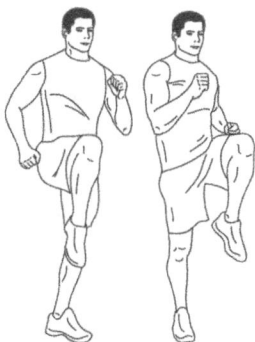

20sec high knees   **20sec** plank hold   **20sec** high knees

32   Good Morning Yoga

Mind and body, working together create an unstoppable combination making you healthier, more focused and stronger. This foundation is built incrementally with small, measured steps which is where Good Morning Yoga workout comes in. Designed to help you meet each and every day on your terms, this is the kind of workout that changes you inside and out.

Focus: Wellbeing

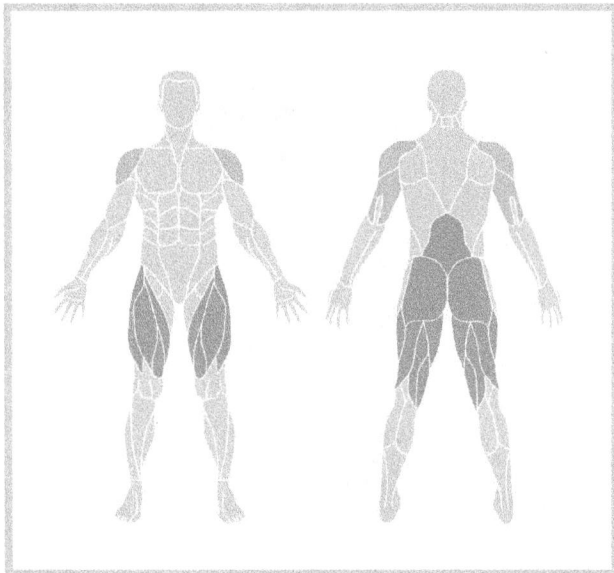

GOOD MORNING
YOGA

BY DAREBEE
ⓒ darebee.com
Hold each pose
for **30 seconds**
then move on
to the next one.

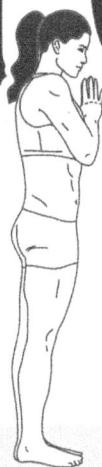

1. mountain pose

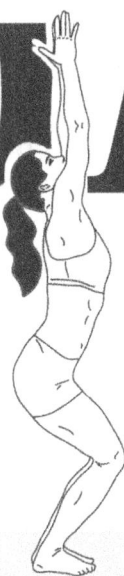

2. fierce pose

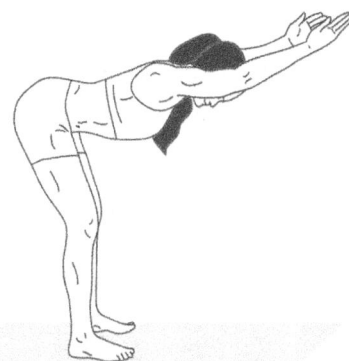

3. forward bend

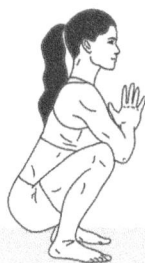

4. wide squat pose

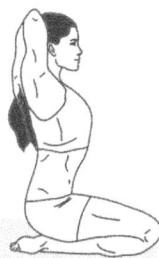

5. hero pose

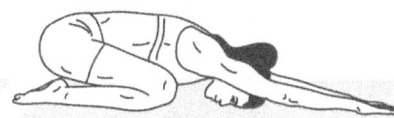

6. child pose

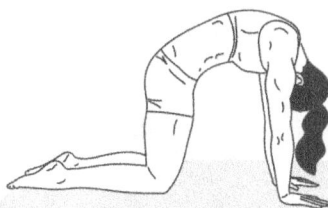

7. cat pose

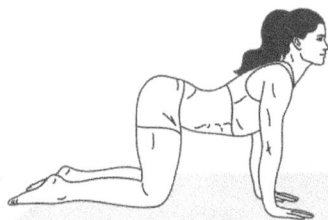

8. cow pose

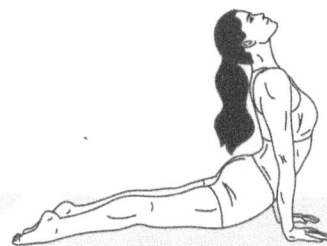

9. upward dog pose

Grit & Grace

As the title suggests - this workout helps you develop grit and grace through endurance and agility exercises combined in a single circuit. Keep your pace steady during jumping jacks, speed up and go all out during pacer steps and mind your form during squat hold, deadlifts and side leg raises. Do half of the reps on one side first and then do the rest on the other.

Focus: High Burn

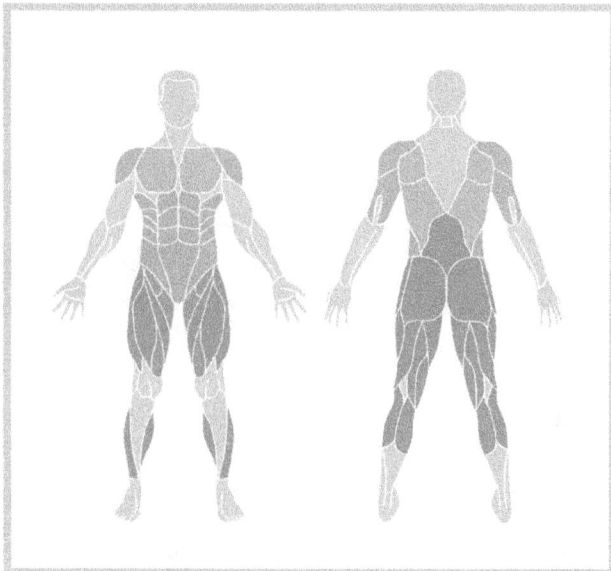

GRIT & GRACE

WORKOUT
BY DAREBEE
© darebee.com

Level I 3 sets
Level II 5 sets
Level III 7 sets
2 minutes rest

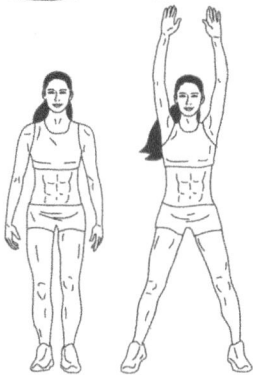

30 jumping jacks

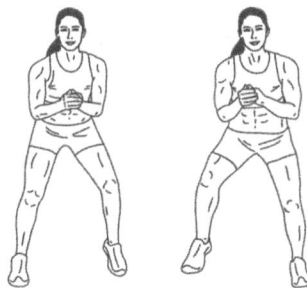

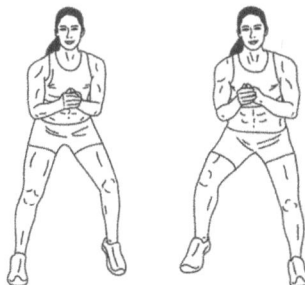

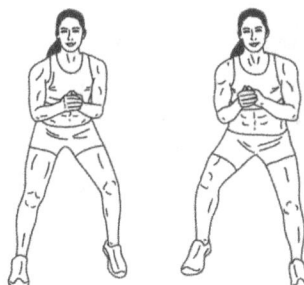

20 pacer steps

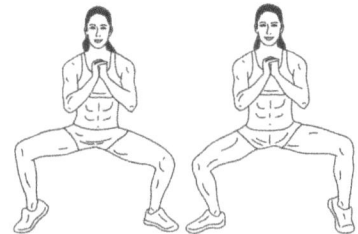

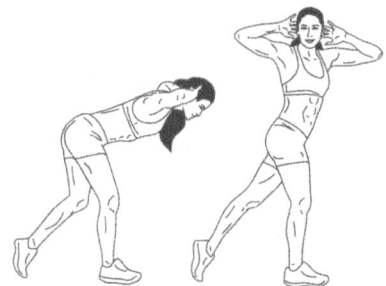

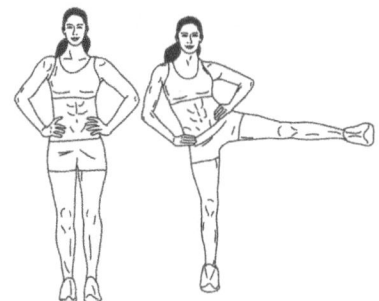

10 squat hold calf raises

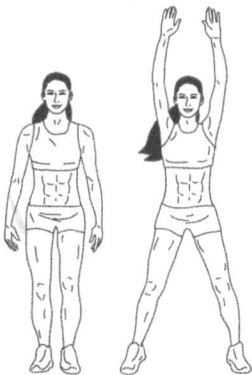

30 jumping jacks

20 pacer steps

10 deadlifts with twist

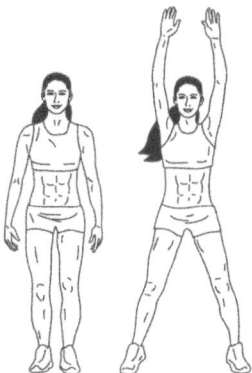

30 jumping jacks

20 pacer steps

10 side leg raises

34 Gut

Exercise creates physical stresses in the body that trigger the adaptive response that changes us physically. The pathway through which this change happens requires hormone signals that activate specific cellular mechanisms. The Gut is a workout that sets you down the path to help your gut bacteria help you get fitter, stronger and healthier.

Focus: High Burn

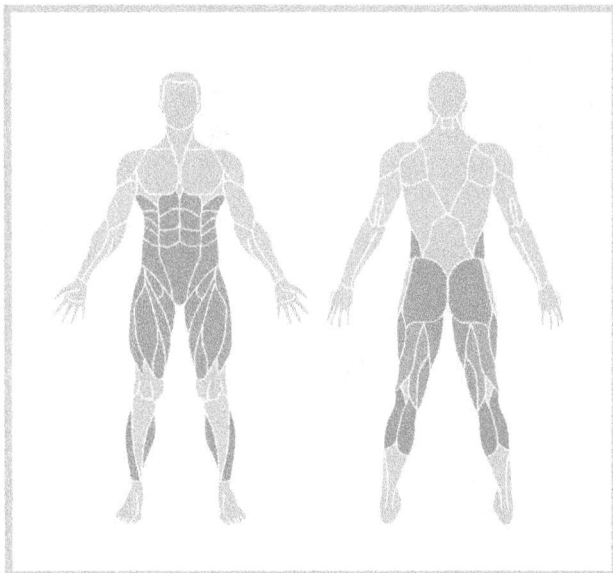

THE GUT

DAREBEE WORKOUT
© darebee.com
Level I 3 sets
Level II 5 sets
Level III 7 sets
2 minutes rest

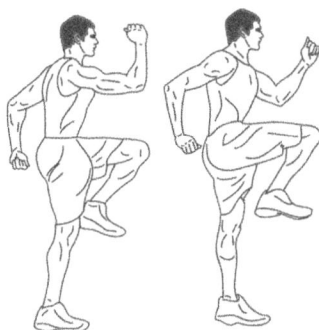

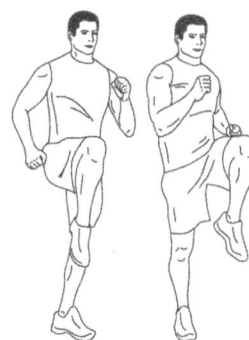

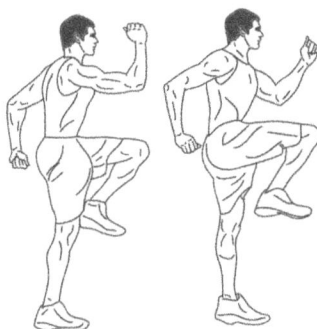

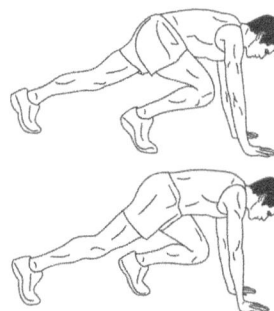

10 march steps
10 high knees

10 march steps
10 climbers

10 march steps
10 knee-to-elbow

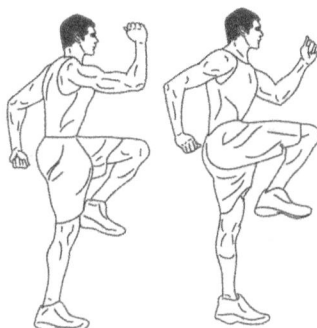

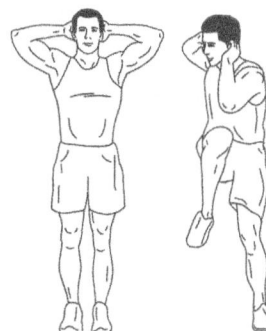

35 Hello, abs!

Strong abs change the performance of every physical activity. They facilitate and preserve power transfer from the lower body to the upper one and vice versa. They affect the way we sit and walk, how quickly we tire and even how explosively we can move. Strong abs require almost daily exercise to develop and maintain. The Hello, Abs! workout is your go-to workout for daily abs exercises. You'll be pleasantly surprised by the results.

Focus: Abs

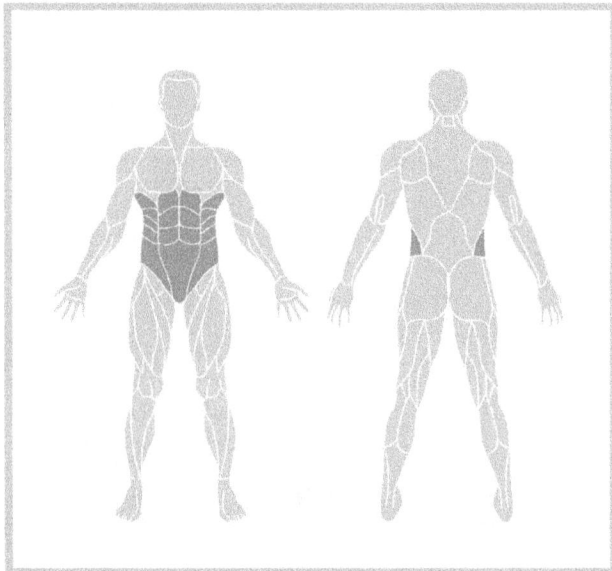

Hello, abs!

DAREBEE WORKOUT © darebee.com

LEVEL I 3 sets **LEVEL II** 4 sets **LEVEL III** 5 sets **REST** up to 2 minutes

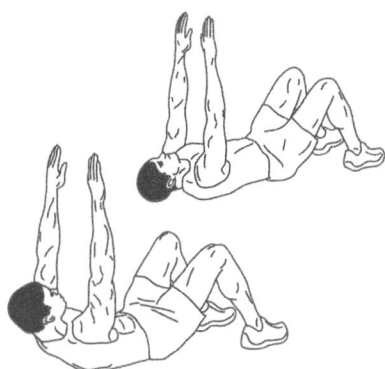

20 high crunches

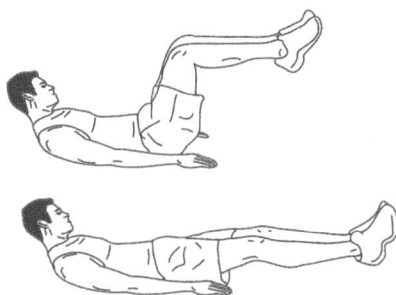

20 crunch kicks

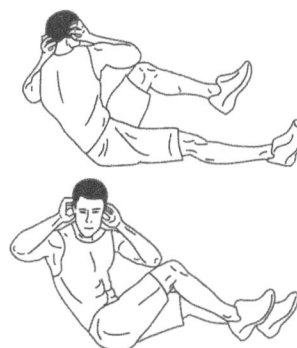

20 knee-to-elbow crunches

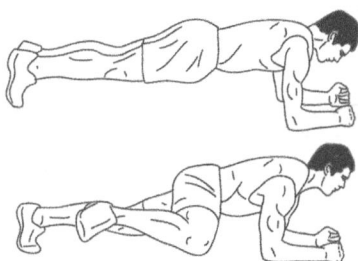

20 plank crunches

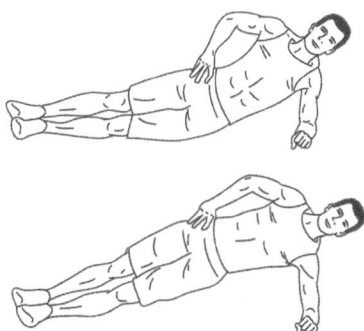

20 side bridges

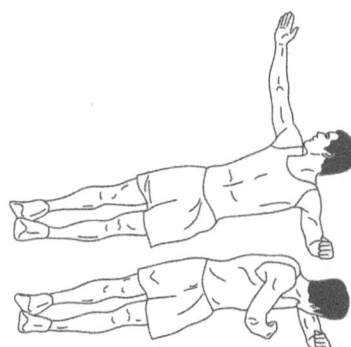

20 side plank rotations

36 Hero

Be your own hero - write your own story! The Hero workout will help you feel stronger, more confident and more in control of your body and your life. Bring your knee all the way to the floor when doing lunges. Go flat out when performing high knees.

Focus: High Burn

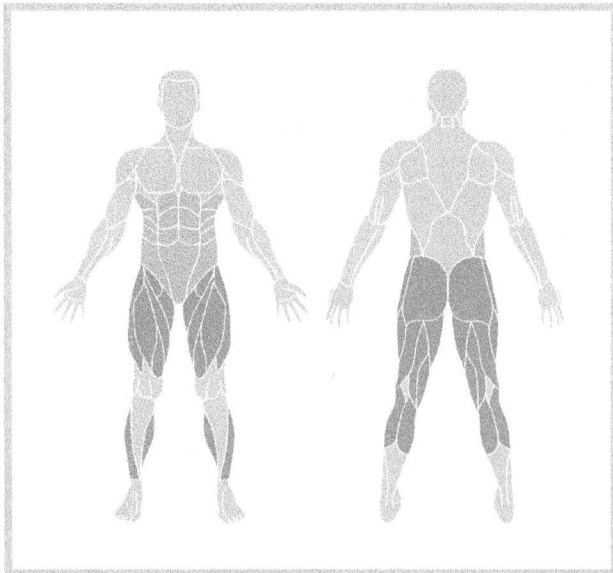

I AM MY OWN HERO

DAREBEE WORKOUT
© darebee.com
Repeat 5 times in total
up to 2 minutes rest in between

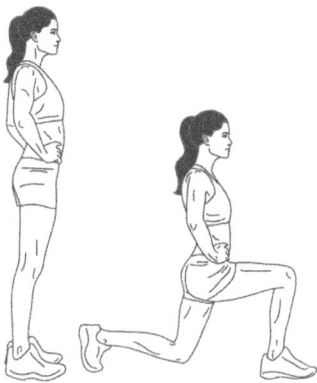

12 lunges

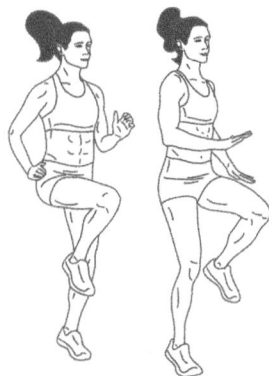

20 high knees

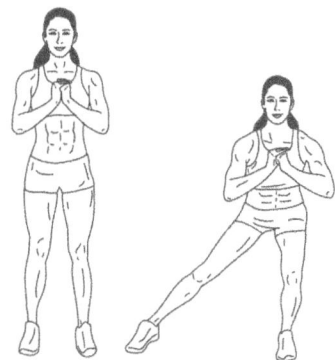

12 side lunges

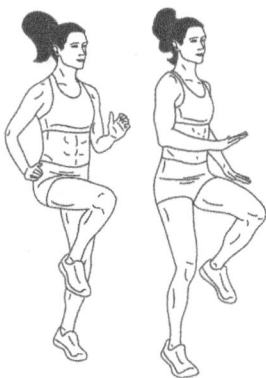

20 high knees

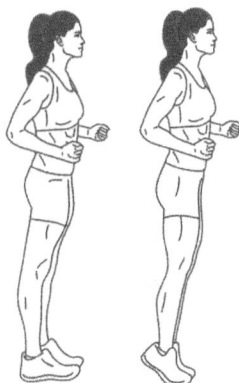

12 calf raises

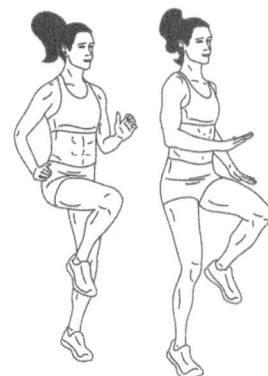

20 high knees

37

Hip Dips

The pelvic area joins the lower body to the upper one and, as such, is key to both the transfer of locomotion and the transport of power from lower body muscles to upper ones (and vice versa). Training it is exactly what Hip Dips is designed to do.

Focus: Strength & Tone

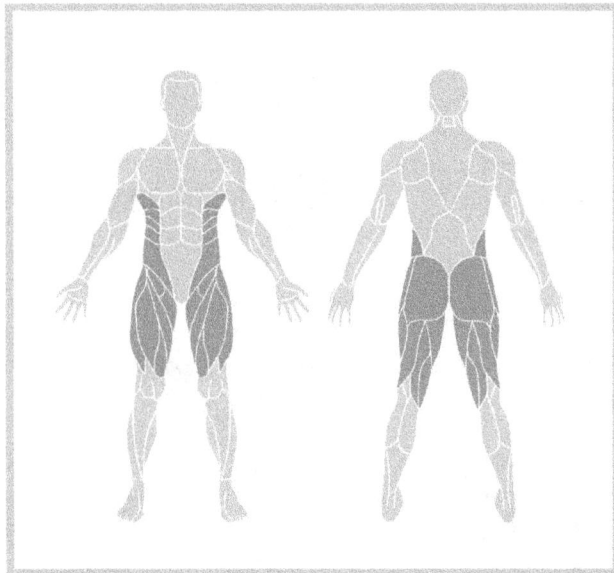

HIP DIPS

DAREBEE WORKOUT © darebee.com

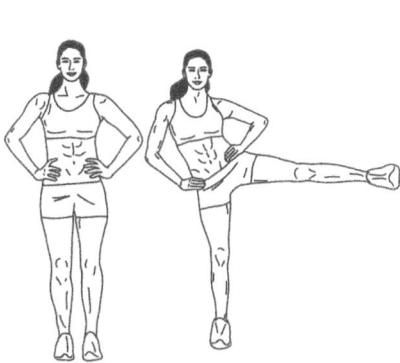

20 side leg raises
x 4 sets in total
20 seconds rest
between sets

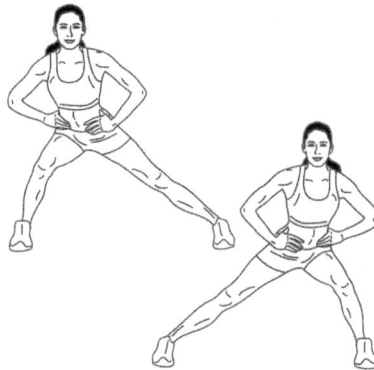

20 side-to-side lunges
x 4 sets in total
20 seconds rest
between sets

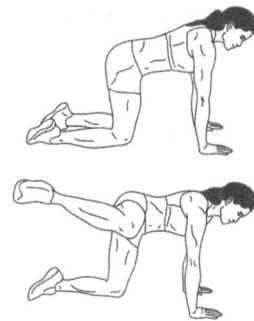

20 side leg extensions
x 4 sets in total
20 seconds rest
between sets

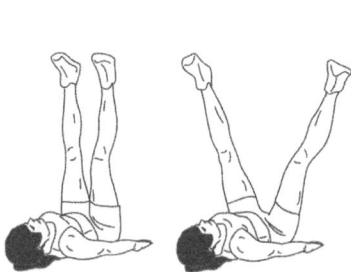

20 V-extensions
x 4 sets in total
20 seconds rest
between sets

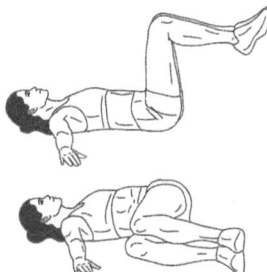

20 half wipers
x 4 sets in total
20 seconds rest
between sets

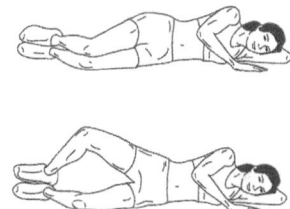

20 clamshells
x 4 sets in total
20 seconds rest
between sets

38

Holistic

The Holistic workout only uses a small set of exercises but each of these uses a large number of muscle groups and attendant satellite muscle groups to produce results in the entire body. If you're looking for a workout that will help you feel strong, capable and awesome then this has to be high on your list.

Focus: Strength & Tone

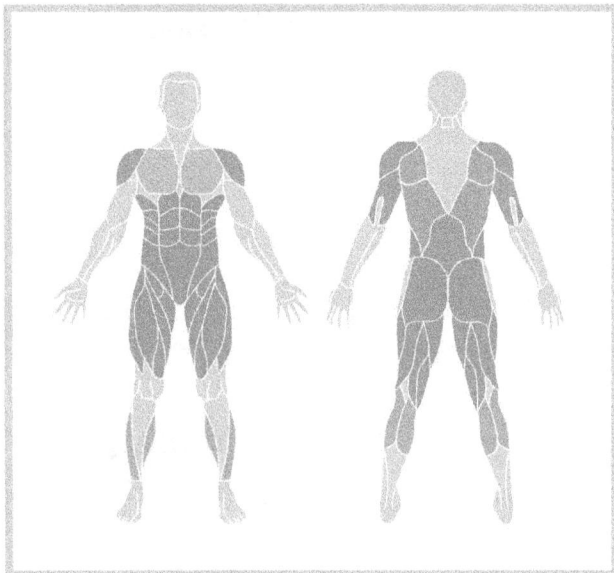

EVERYTHING IS CONNECTED
HOLISTIC

DAREBEE WORKOUT © darebee.com
5 sets | 2 minutes rest between sets

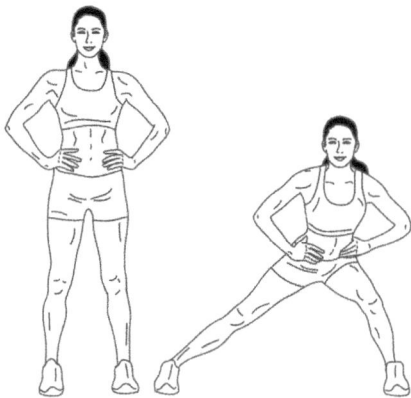

20 side lunges

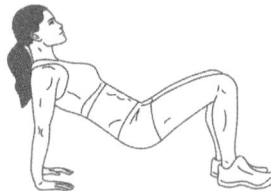

10 tricep dips

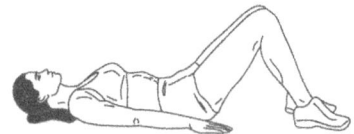

20 bridges

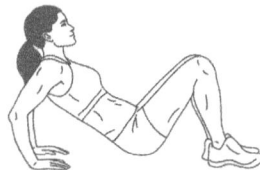

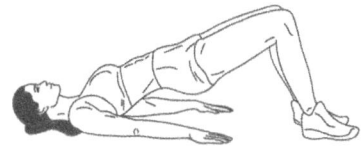

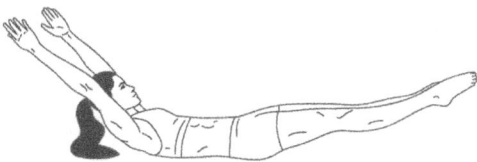

20-count hollow hold

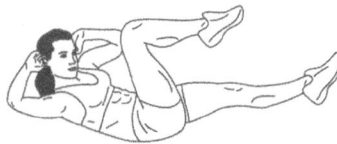

10 knee-to-elbow crunches

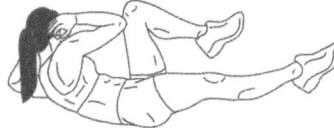

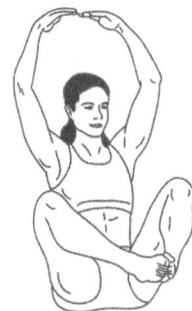

20-count O-pose hold

39 Homemade Abs

Abs need constant work in order to be strong, supple and well-defined. The Homemade Abs workout helps you keep your abs in shape by targeting the four major abdominal muscle groups.

Focus: Abs

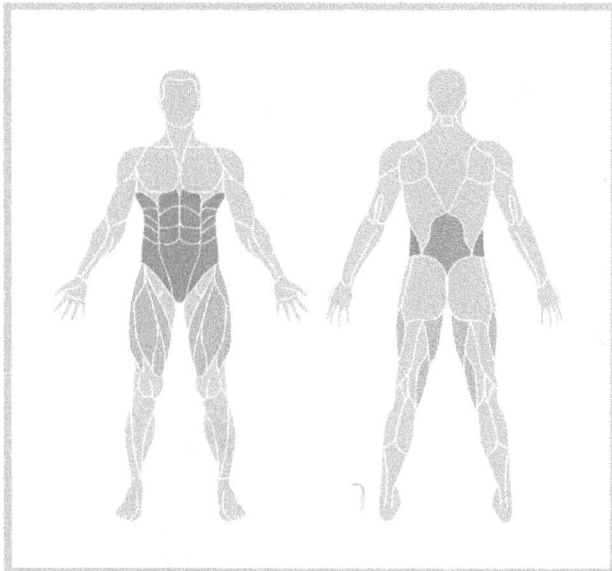

homemade abs

DAREBEE WORKOUT © darebee.com

LEVEL I 3 sets LEVEL II 4 sets LEVEL III 5 sets REST up to 2 minutes

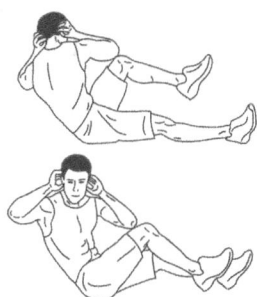

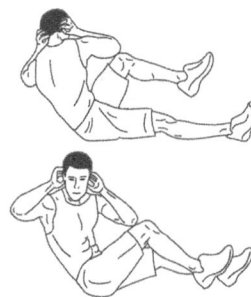

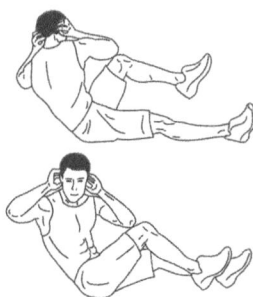

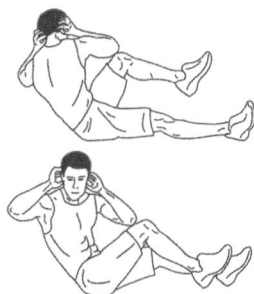

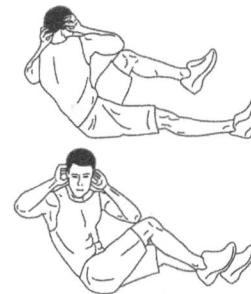

4 knee-to-elbows   **10** leg raises   **4** knee-to-elbows

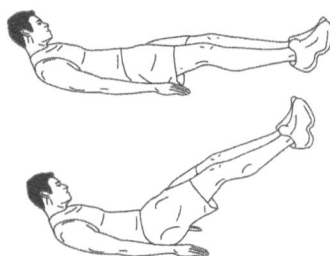

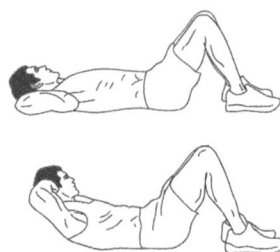

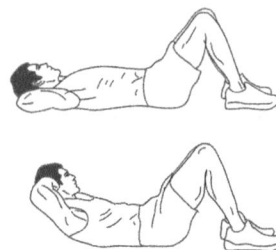

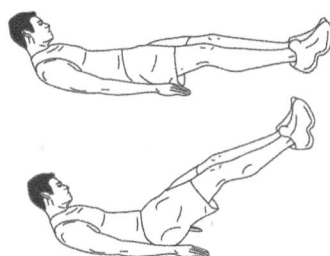

10 crunches   **4** knee-to-elbows   **10** crunches

4 knee-to-elbows   **10** leg raises   **4** knee-to-elbows

40   Homemade Hero

In Homemade Hero you rest by training your core, which means that during the more active part of this HIIT workout you really need to up the intensity and get the numbers in, even if it means reducing the quality of your form. The benefits are stronger, leaner muscles and an aerobic system that will let you catch the bus every time you run for it.

Focus: High Knees

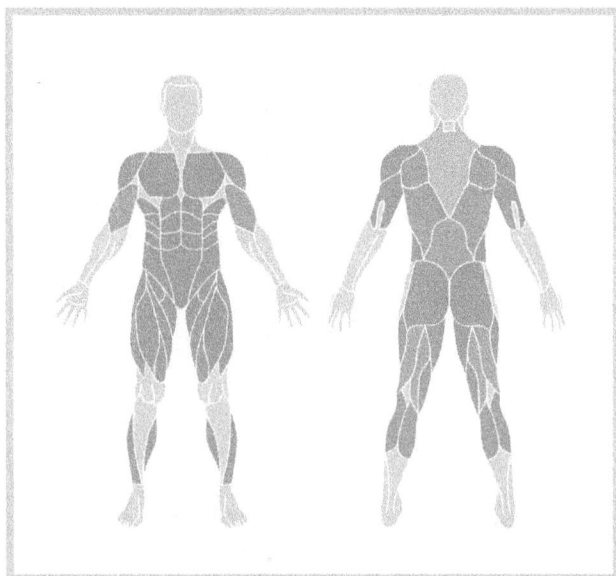

HOMEMADE HERO

DAREBEE HIIT WORKOUT
© darebee.com
Level I 3 sets
Level II 5 sets
Level III 7 sets
2 minutes rest

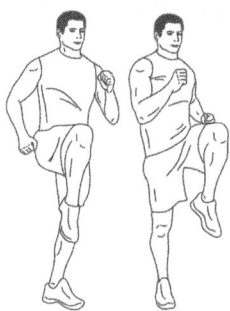

20sec high knees

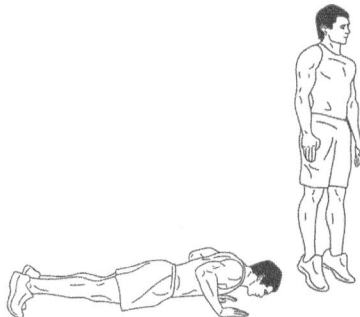

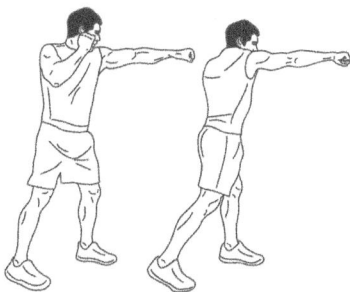

20sec burpees

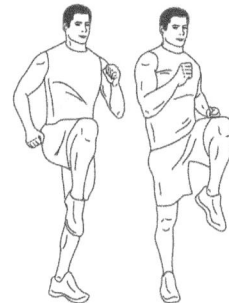

20sec high knees

20sec punches

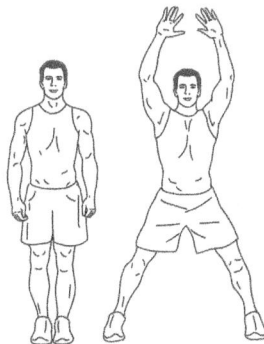

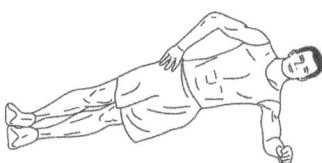

20sec jumping jacks

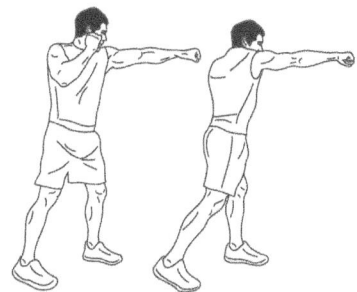

20sec punches

20sec side plank (right)

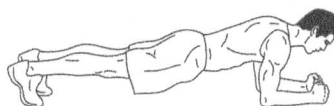

20sec elbow plank

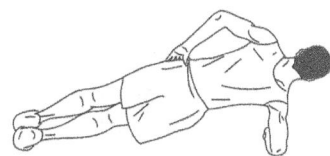

20sec side plank (left)

41 Huff & Puff

When it comes to HIIT speed and rep count are important because they help maintain intensity and it's intensity that delivers results. So, really, for Huff & Puff as for all of the High Intensity Interval Training workouts you want to start as fast and hard as you can, improve on it after the first set or two and then maintain the intensity by keeping track of the rep count for each exercise. That way you're really pushing against the edges of your ability and forcing your body to improve.

Focus: High Knees

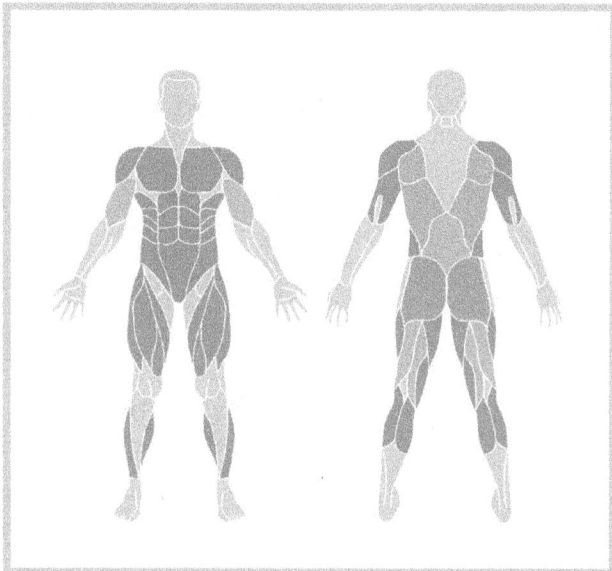

HUFF & PUFF

DAREBEE HIIT WORKOUT © darebee.com

Level I 3 sets **Level II** 5 sets **Level III** 7 sets | 2 minutes rest

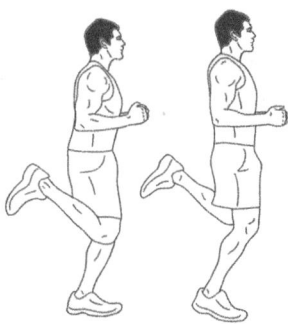

20sec butt kicks

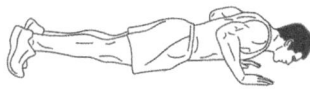

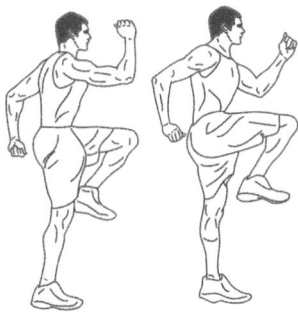

20sec push-up plank hold

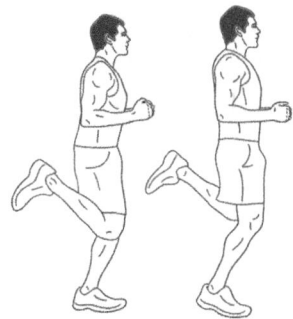

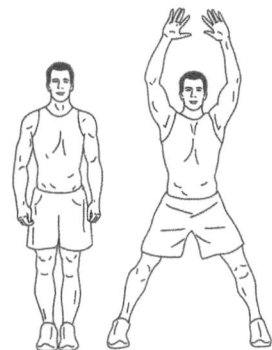

20sec butt kicks

20sec march steps

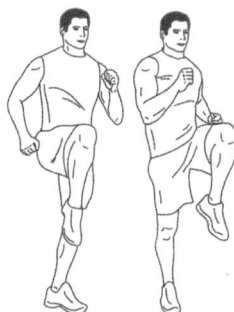

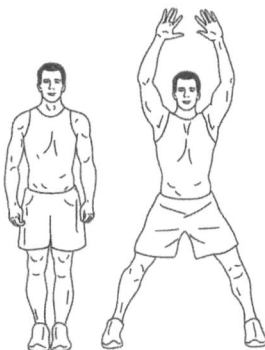

20sec high knees

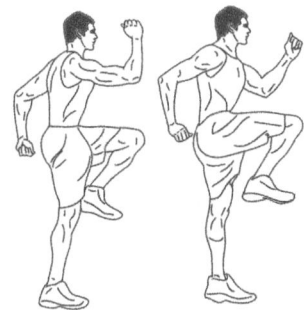

20sec march steps

20sec jumping jacks

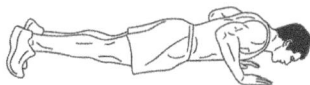

20sec push-up plank hold

20sec jumping jacks

Inquisitor

Some workouts should come with a warning. The Inquisitor makes some pretty hefty demands in the body's ability to recruit and then coordinate large muscle groups, fascial strength, tendons and satellite muscle groups in order to generate controlled power. The result is a workout that is definitely not for beginners, but it should be in your exercise event horizon.

Focus: High Burn

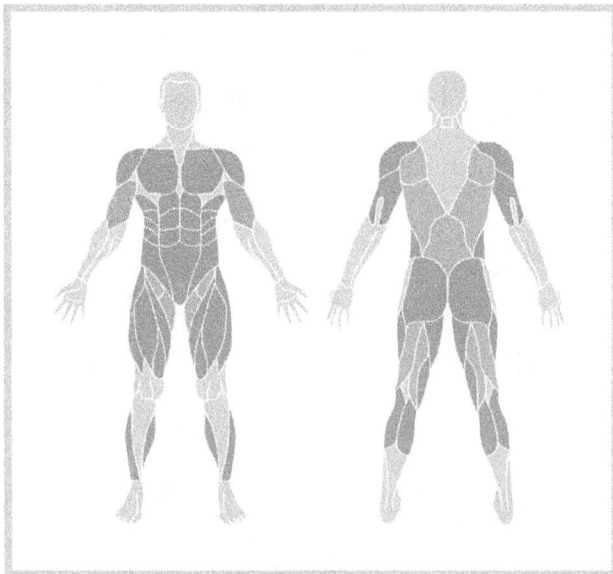

INQUISITOR

DAREBEE WORKOUT © darebee.com

LEVEL I 3 sets **LEVEL II** 5 sets **LEVEL III** 7 sets **REST** up to 2 minutes

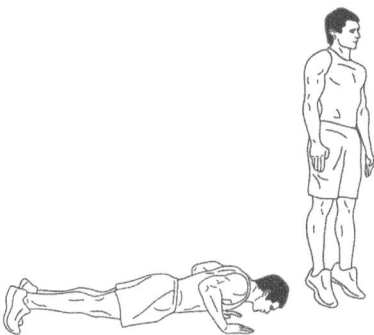

10 burpees

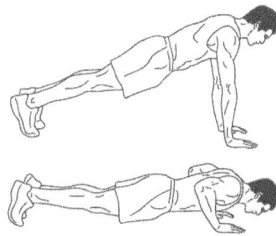

10 push-ups

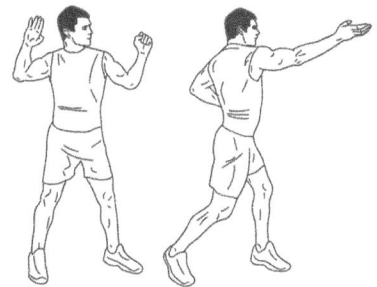

20 knife hand strikes

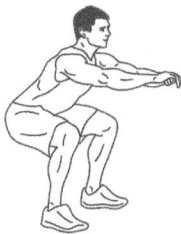

10-count squat hold

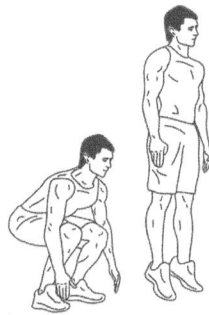

10 jump squats

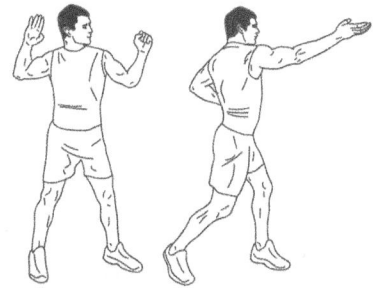

20 knife hand strikes

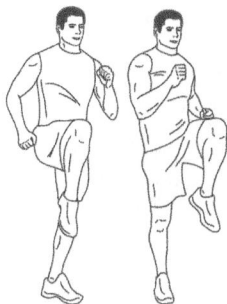

10 high knees

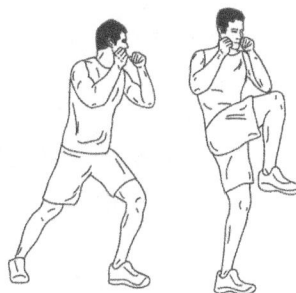

10 knee strikes

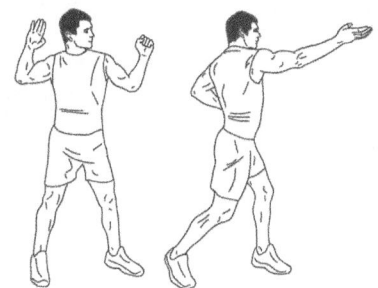

20 knife hand strikes

43 Into The Fire

Combining a number of gravity-fighting moves and combat moves Into The Fire is a workout designed to challenge strength, endurance and coordination. This is a difficulty Level IV workout which means it's not really suitable for those who are new to fitness or for those coming back in from a long lay-off, but it should definitely be on your horizon.

Focus: High Knees

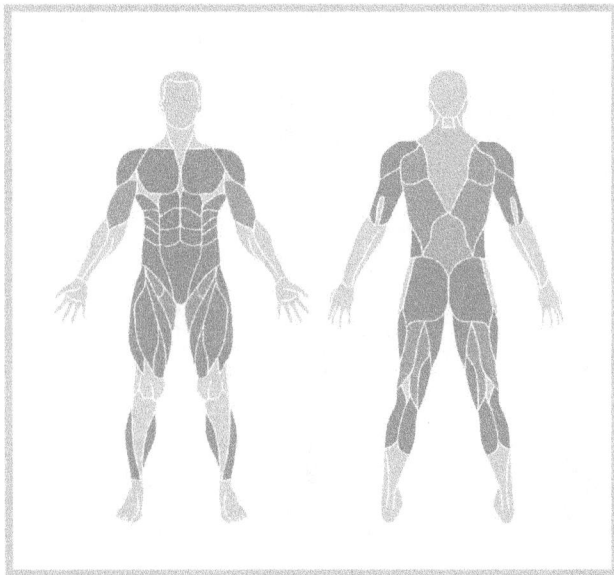

INTO THE FIRE

DAREBEE HIIT WORKOUT © darebee.com

Level I 3 sets **Level II** 5 sets **Level III** 7 sets | 2 minutes rest

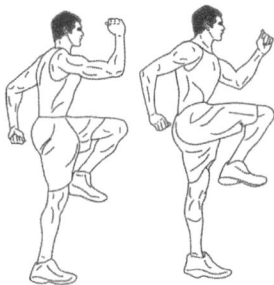

30sec march steps

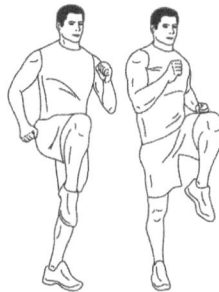

15sec high knees

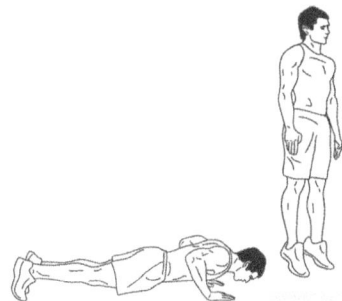

15sec burpees

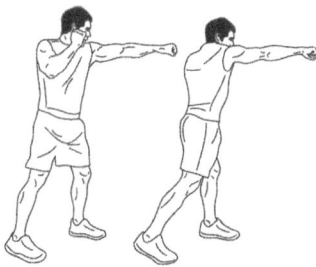

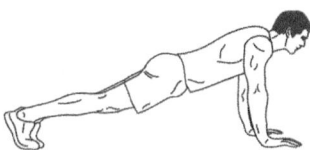

30sec punches

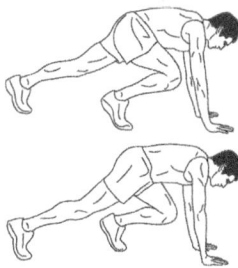

15sec climbers

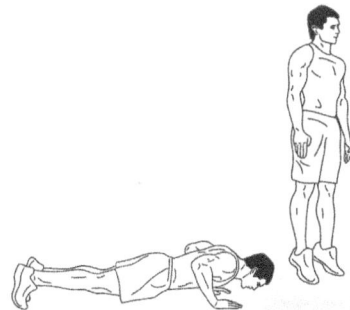

15sec burpees

30sec plank hold

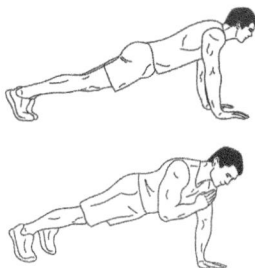

15sec shoulder taps

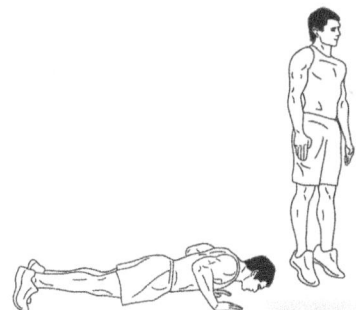

15sec burpees

44 Lady Knight

Awaken the warrior inside with the Lady Knight Workout. Go slow and focus on form for this one - make sure your knee almost reaches the floor when performing lunges.

Focus: Strength & Tone

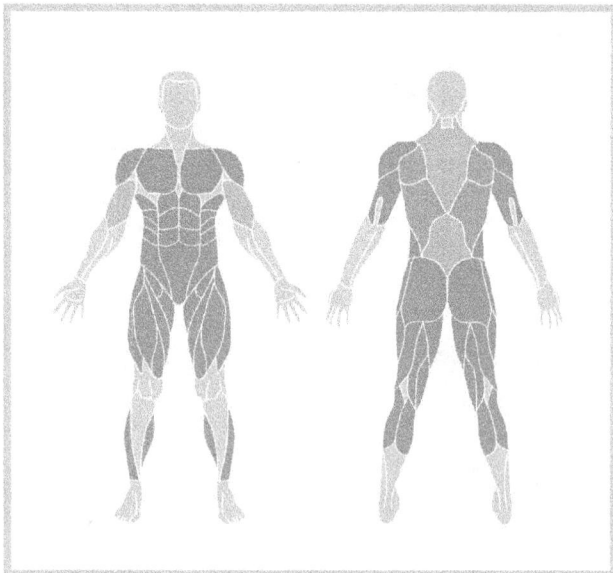

Lady Knight

DAREBEE WORKOUT
© darebee.com
Level I   3 sets
Level II 5 sets
Level III 7 sets
2 minutes rest

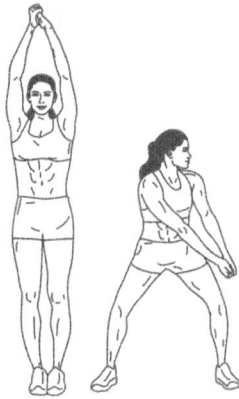

20 cross chops

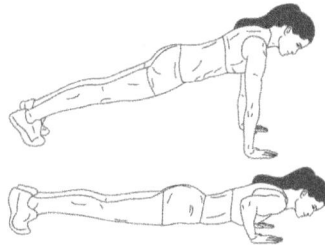

6 push-ups

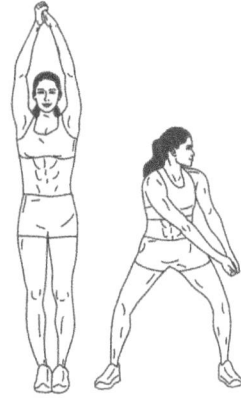

20 cross chops

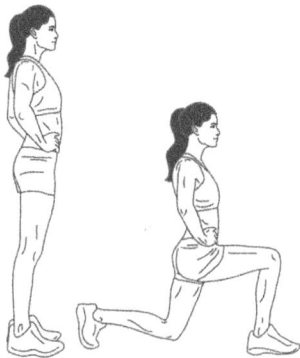

6 lunges

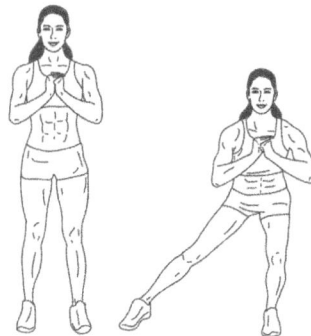

6 side lunges

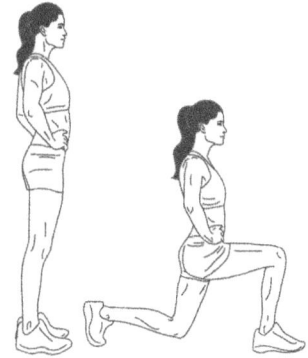

6 lunges

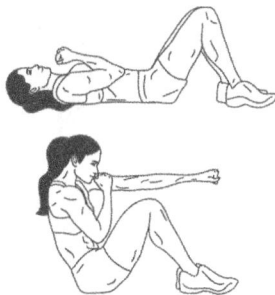

6 sit-up punches

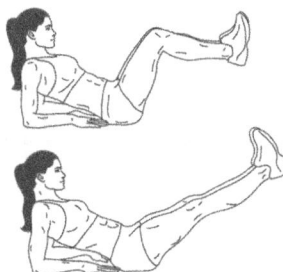

6 crunch kicks

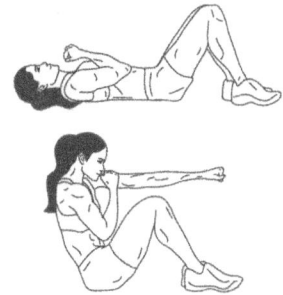

6 sit-up punches

45 Lean & Mean

There are a few things you need to get lean: a high-burn workout that will work large muscle groups, force you to use up a lot of oxygen and get you into the sweatzone fast. Exercises that keep on applying a load to your muscles. And a combination that forces you to recruit a large number of muscle groups. Lean and Mean combines all that. You now just need to power through it. Maintain perfect form.

Focus: High Burn

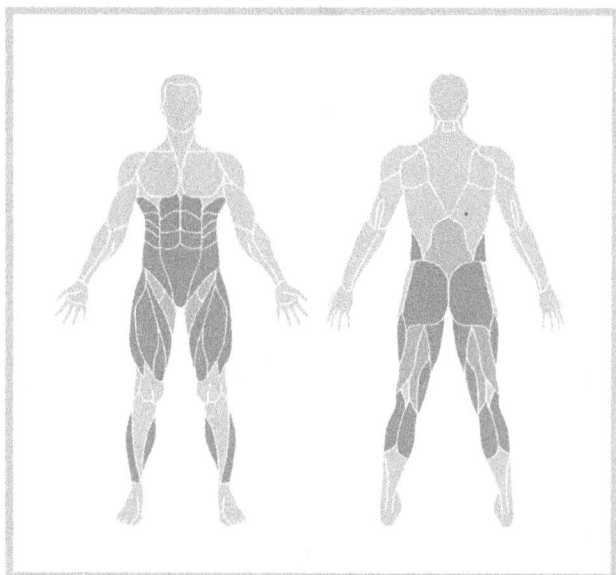

LEAN &MEAN

DAREBEE WORKOUT © darebee.com

LEVEL I 3 sets **LEVEL II** 5 sets **LEVEL III** 7 sets **REST** up to 2 minutes

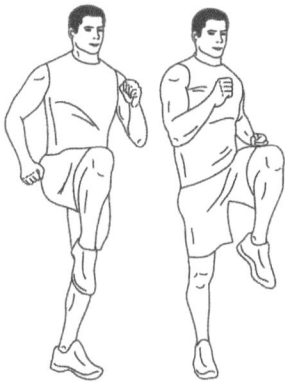

40 high knees

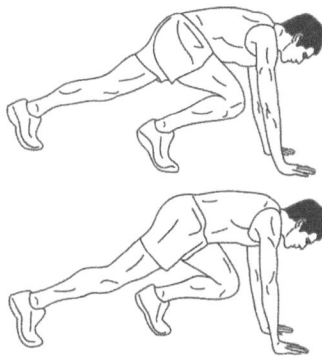

40 climbers

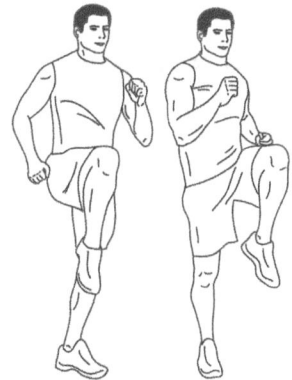

40 high knees

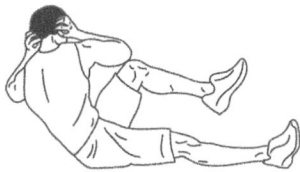

20 knee-to-elbows

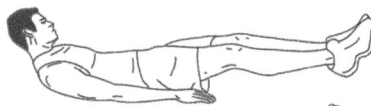

20 leg raises

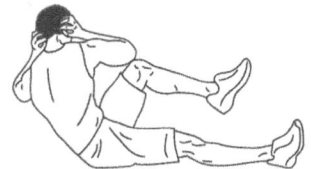

20 knee-to-elbows

46   Live Long

We now know that exercise is key to a longer and healthier life. To live long and, hopefully, prosper add a minimum of 15 minutes of cardiovascular exercise to your day. It all adds up and eventually makes a big difference in how you look and feel. Go through the circuit as fast as you can, catch your breath and go again.

Focus: Strength & Tone

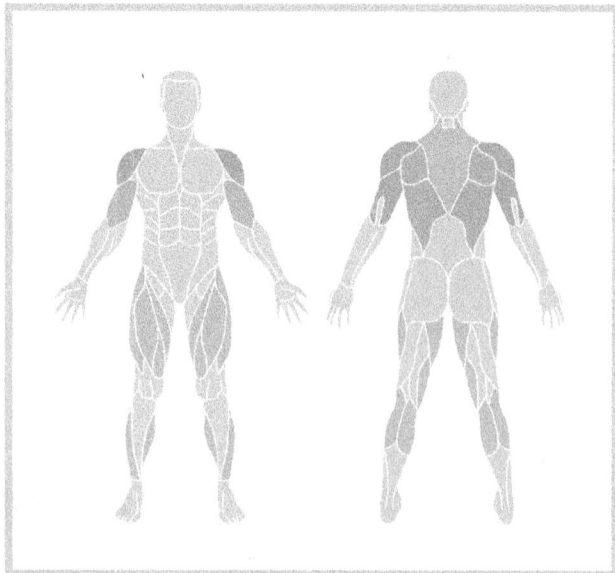

LIVE LONG

DAREBEE WORKOUT
© darebee.com

Level I 3 sets
Level II 5 sets
Level III 7 sets
2 minutes rest

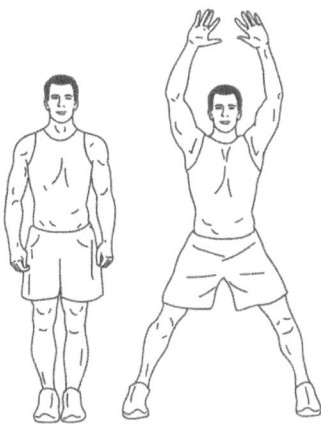

10 jumping jacks

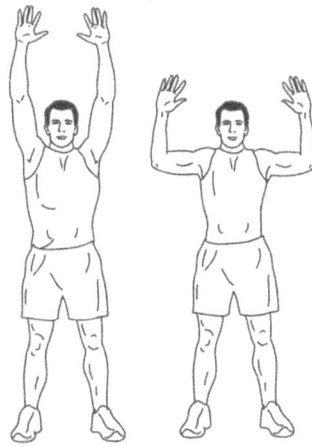

20 standing W-extensions

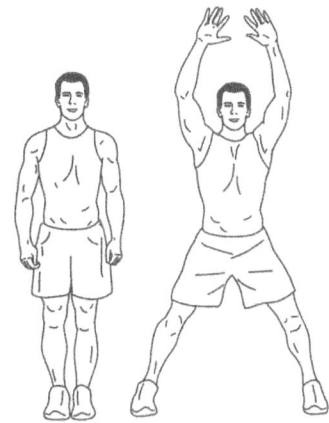

10 jumping jacks

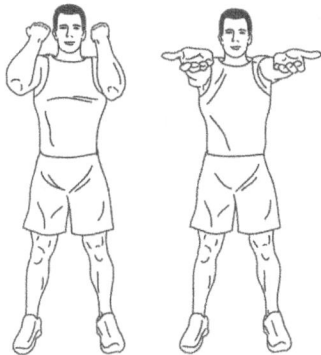

20 bicep extensions

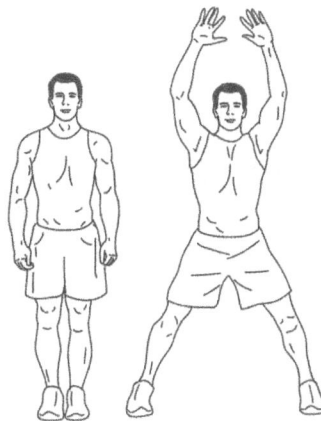

10 jumping jacks

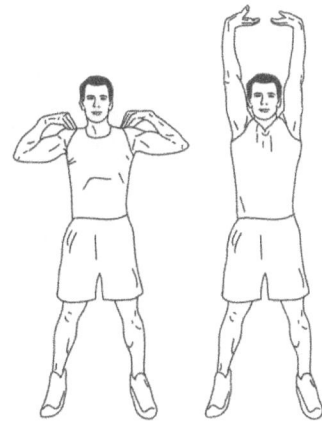

20 shoulder taps

47 Lunch

Earn Your Lunch is a quick but intense workout you can literally do before your lunch (or during your lunch break). The best part? You will only need 10 minutes in total (including breaks!). It's guaranteed to make you work for your meal. You can go at your own pace but - if you can and the environment allows it - go flat out!

Focus: High Burn

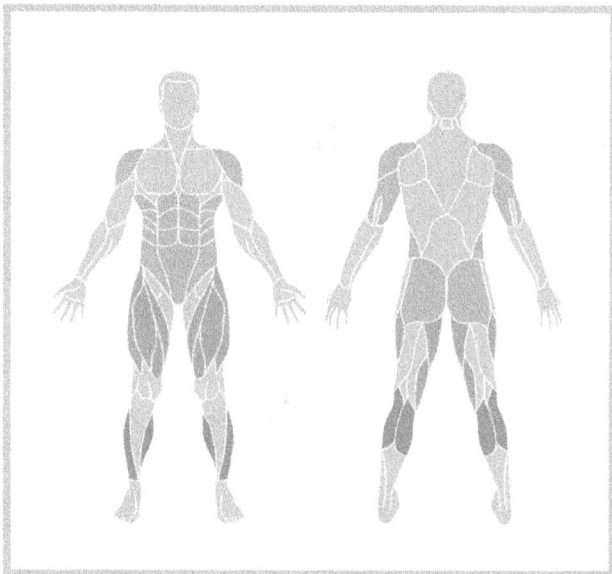

EARN YOUR LUNCH WORKOUT

by DAREBEE © darebee.com

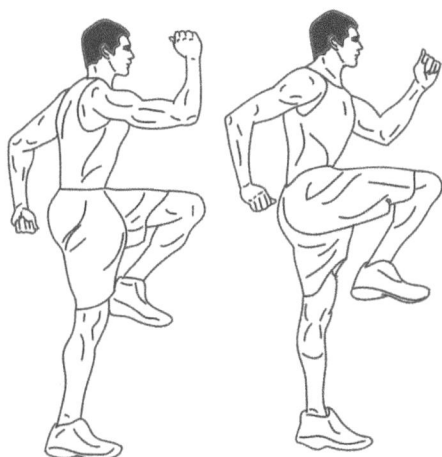

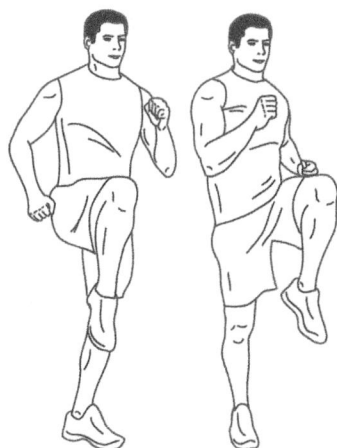

1 minute march steps (warmup)

1 minute high knees

1 minute rest

1 minute high knees

1 minute rest

1 minute high knees

1 minute rest

1 minute high knees

1 minute rest

1 minute high knees

done

48 Make My Day

If you want to move fast, change directions quickly, fight with devastating effectiveness, then you need to either relocate to a planet with a lower gravity or reduce the mass of your body, effectively making yourself lighter. The Make My Day workout does just that, by making you feel lighter. Successive exercise spit your bodyweight against gravity and you end up gasping for breath. This is not suitable for beginners. Then again if you got reading this far, you're most probably not a beginner.

Focus: High Burn

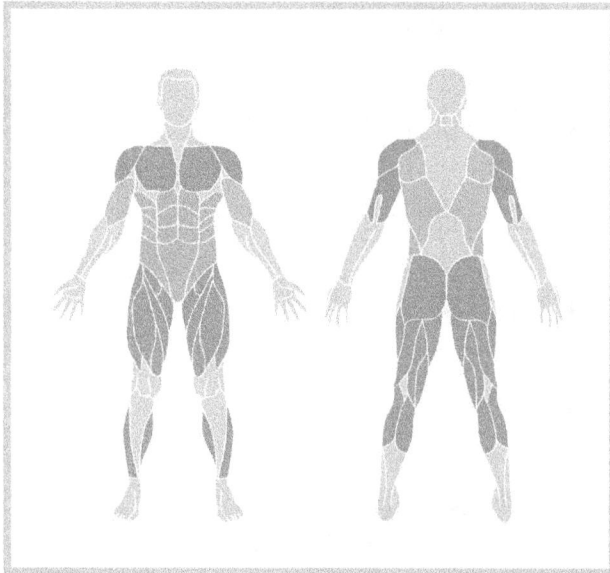

GO AHEAD
MAKE MY DAY

DAREBEE WORKOUT
© darebee.com

LEVEL I 3 sets
LEVEL II 5 sets
LEVEL III 7 sets
REST up to 2 minutes

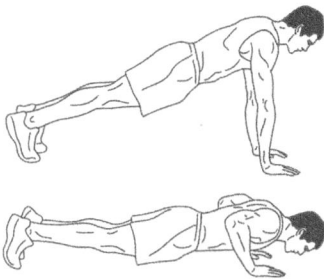

10 push-ups

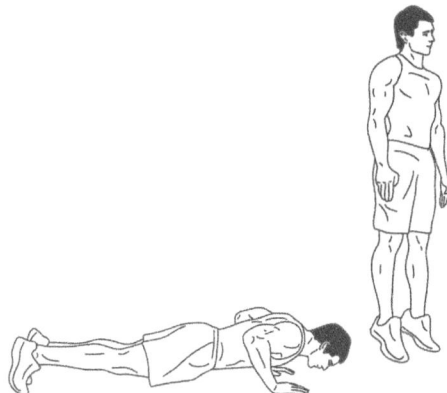

10 burpees

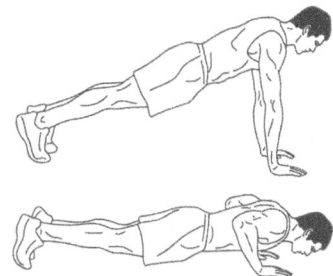

10 push-ups

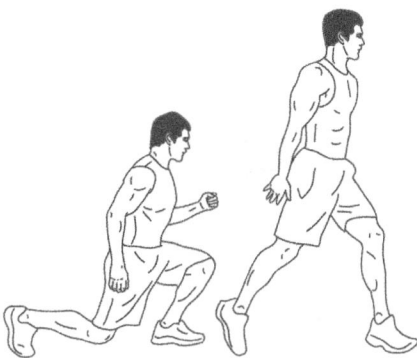

10 jumping lunges

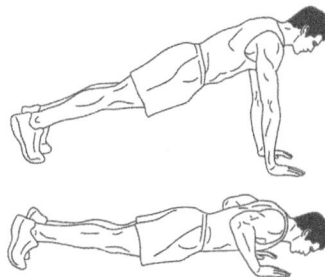

10 push-ups

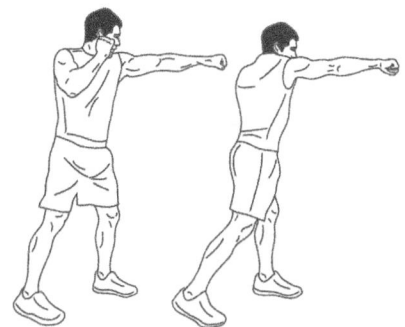

30 punches

Micro Shred

Abs are there to be worked frequently, at an accessible level. Micro Shred is only a difficulty Level II workout but add it to the routines you go to when you're not busy discovering the limits of your physical capability and feel the difference it will make to your basic abs and core strength.

Focus: Abs

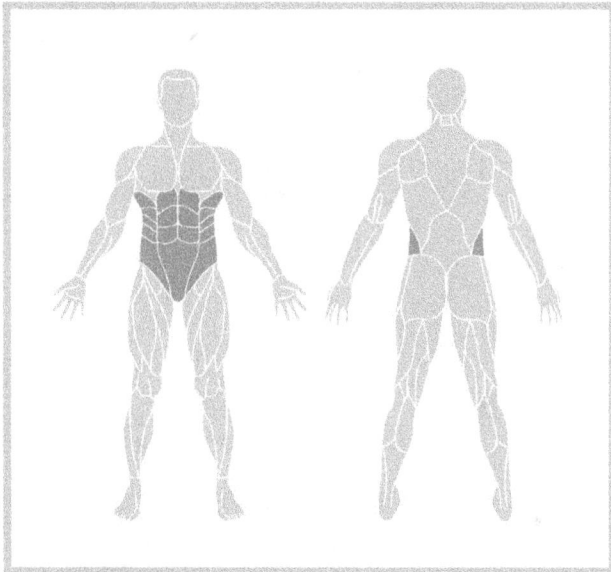

MICRO SHRED

WORKOUT by DAREBEE © darebee.com

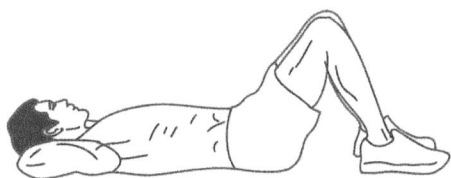
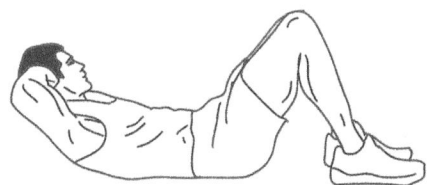
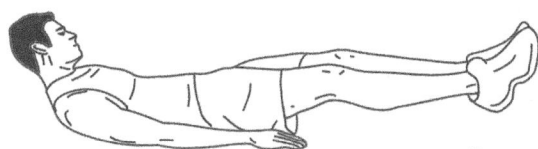
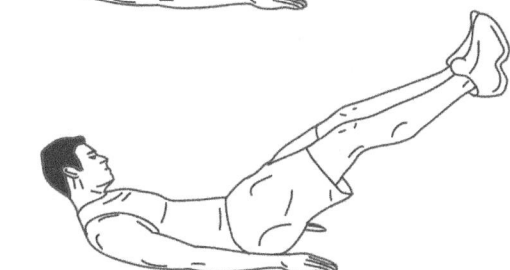

20 crunches

10 leg raises

20 crunches

10 leg raises

20 crunches

10 leg raises

20 crunches

10 leg raises

20 crunches

10 leg raises

done

50 Monkey!

Get your Monkey on! Crawl, jump and kick as if you were trapped under a mountain for 500 years. Liberate your body and your muscles and get back into action. Try to go from climbers to burpees and back to climbers on the fly, with no pauses.

Focus: Combat

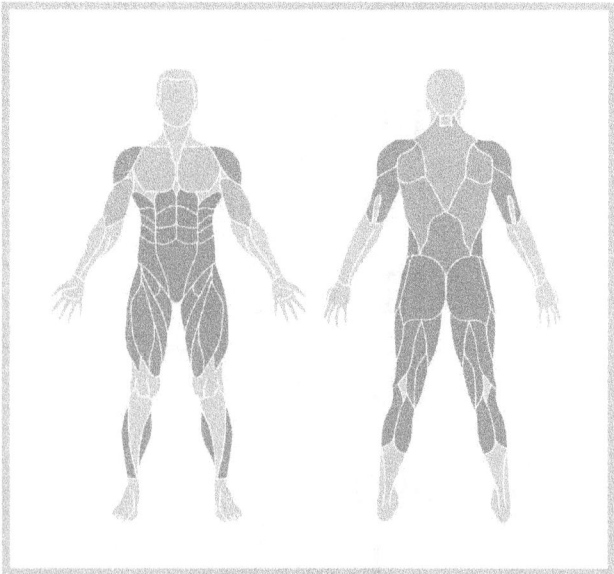

MONKEY!

DAREBEE WORKOUT © darebee.com

LEVEL I 3 sets **LEVEL II** 5 sets **LEVEL III** 7 sets **REST** up to 2 minutes

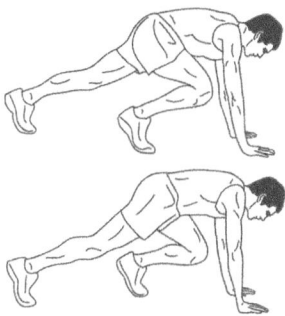

10 climbers

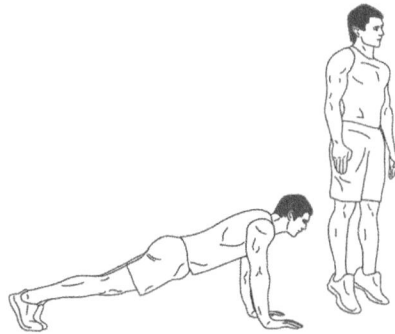

10 basic burpees

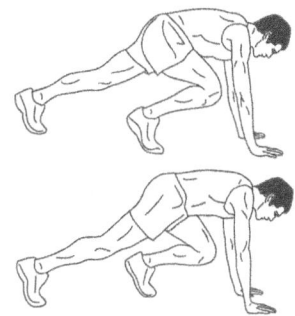

10 climbers

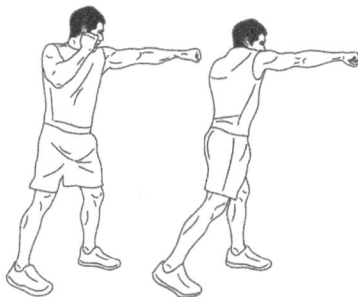

20 punches

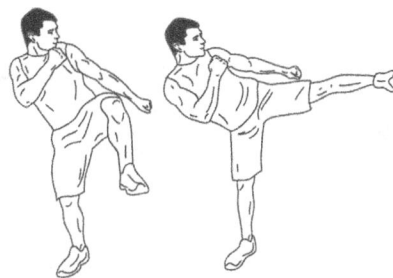

20 side kicks

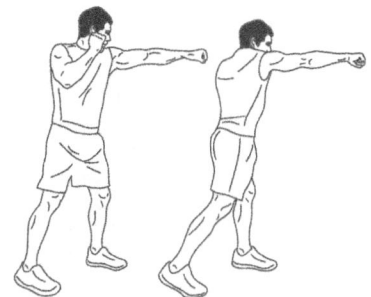

20 punches

51 Monster Inside

Monster Inside is a strength workout that leverages the body's own weight to produce a set of exercises designed to work virtually every muscle of the body bar the back. On days when you don't feel like anything other than a workout that helps you hone your physical strength and creates the basis for further progress this is the perfect exercise routine to go for.

Focus: Strength & Tone

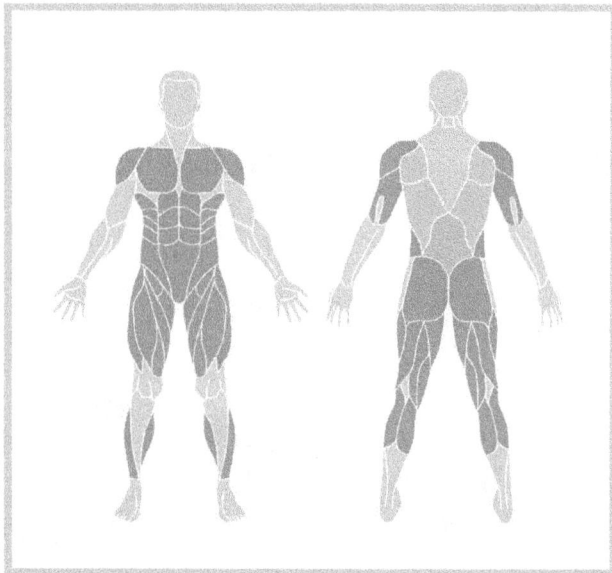

MONSTER INSIDE

DAREBEE WORKOUT © darebee.com

2 minutes rest between exercises

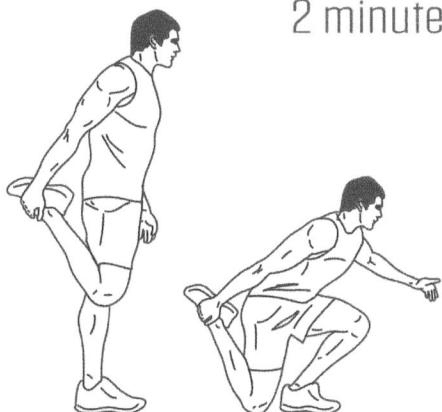

20 shrimp squats **x 3 sets** in total
20 seconds rest between sets

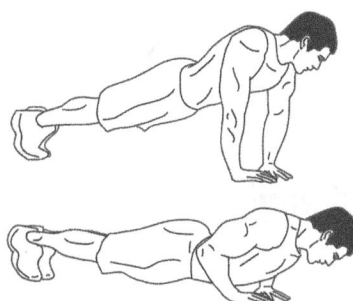

12 close grip push-ups
x 3 sets in total | 20 seconds rest

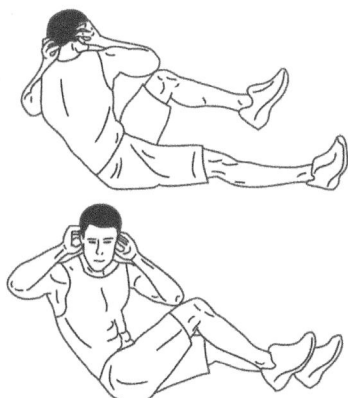

20 knee-to-elbow crunches
x 3 sets in total | 20 seconds rest

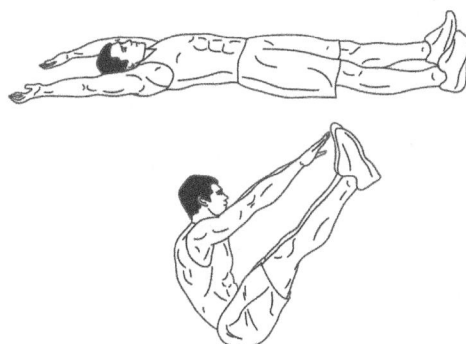

12 V-ups **x 3 sets** in total
20 seconds rest between sets

52

Morning Stretch

Stretching helps conditions tendons and muscles, increases flexibility, can prevent injury and actually leads to greater strength. The Morning Stretch workout is one of those 'little' routines that help you become unstoppable and stay that way.

Focus: Wellbeing

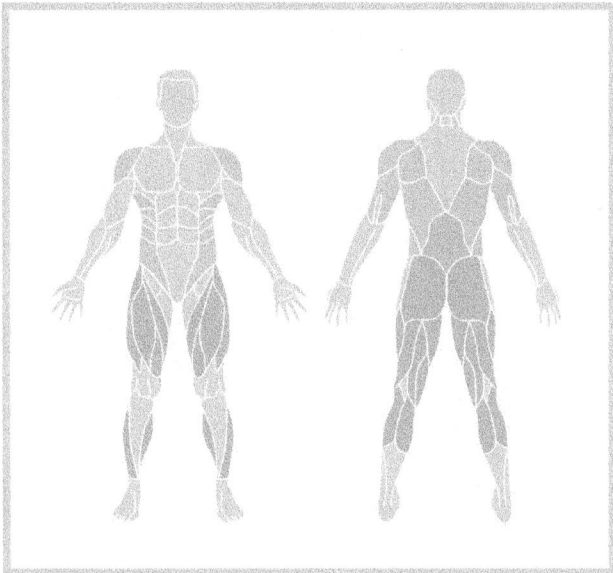

morning
stretch

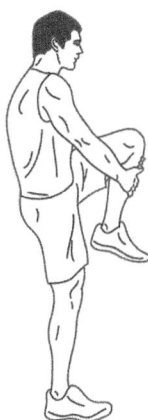

by DAREBEE
© darebee.com
30 seconds each

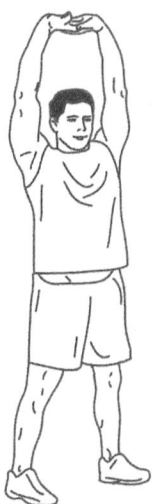

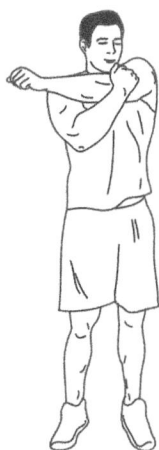

shoulder stretch #1   shoulder stretch #2   upper back stretch   core stretch

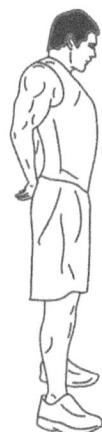

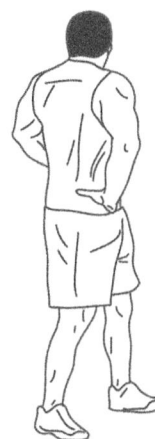

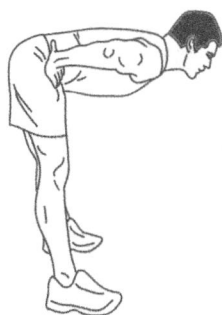

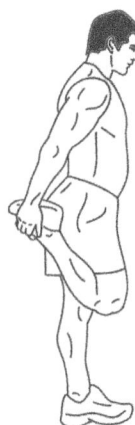

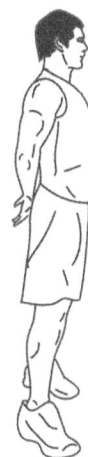

hamstring stretch   glute stretch   quad stretch   calf raise hold

53

Nix

If you're ready to test your lung capacity, aerobic fitness, recovery rate and endurance then welcome to The Nix workout. Moving large muscle groups, explosively, many times is a guarantee to use up any on-board fuel stored in the muscles and the bloodstream and activate the Krebs Cycle to give you a satisfying burn. This is a difficulty Level V workout which means that it's not really suitable for beginners. But it is definitely the kind of workout you want to own some day.

Focus: High Knees

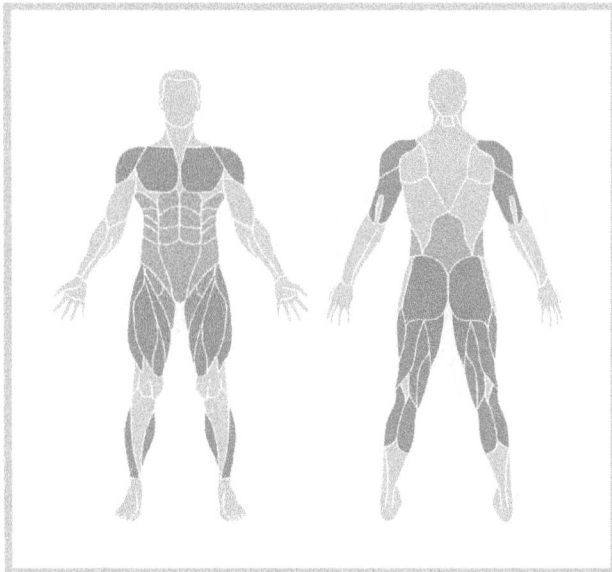

The Nix

DAREBEE WORKOUT © darebee.com

LEVEL I 3 sets **LEVEL II** 5 sets **LEVEL III** 7 sets **REST** up to 2 minutes

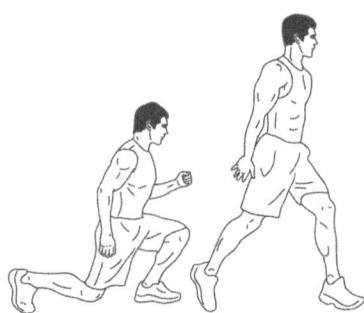

20 jumping lunges

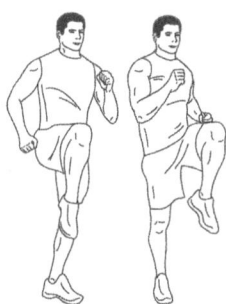

40 high knees

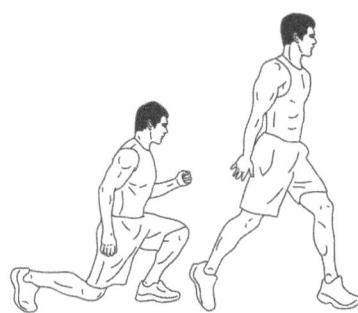

20 jumping lunges

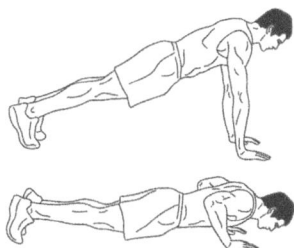

20 push-ups

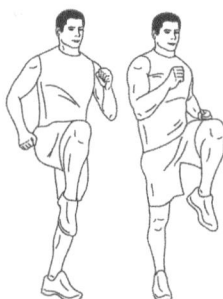

40 high knees

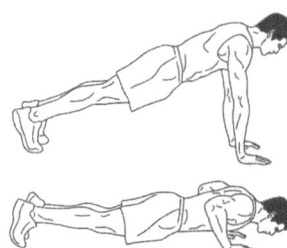

20 push-ups

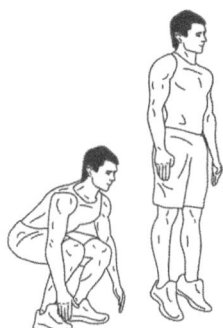

20 jump squats

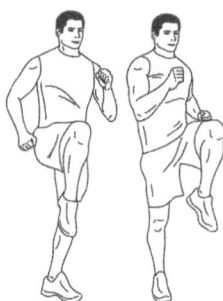

40 high knees

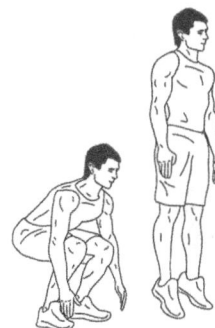

20 jump squats

54 No Surrender

You know that the moment you get a workout called No Surrender it's really a challenge because surrender is what you'd want to do. Resist the fatigue that's designed to build up and maintain your output throughout each set. This one's all about the intensity.

Focus: High Burn

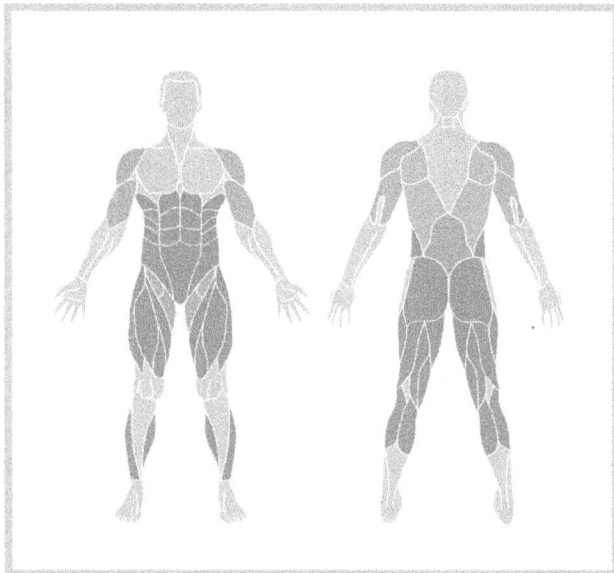

NO SURRENDER

DAREBEE HIIT WORKOUT © darebee.com

Level I 3 sets **Level II** 5 sets **Level III** 7 sets | 2 minutes rest

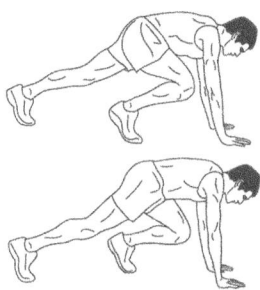

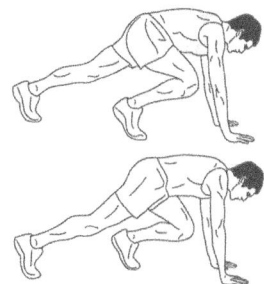

20sec climbers **20sec** high knees **20sec** climbers

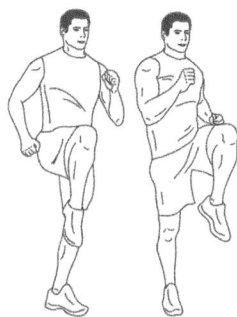

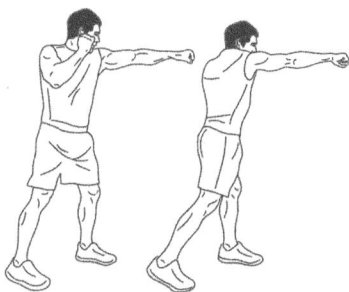

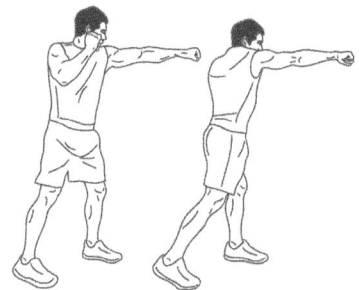

20sec punches **20sec** high knees **20sec** punches

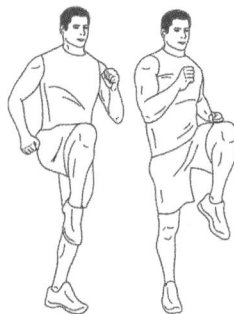

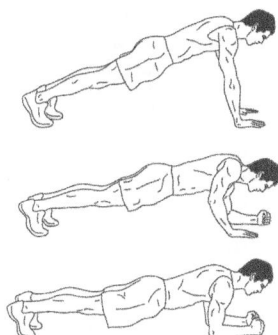

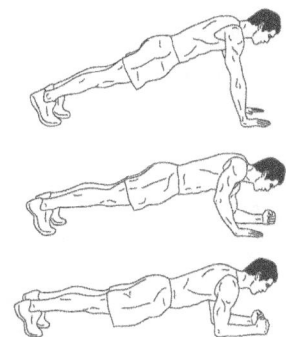

20sec up & down planks **20sec** high knees **20sec** up & down planks

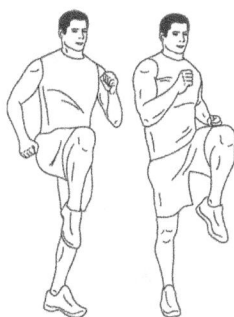

55 Odyssey

The Odyssey took ten years to deliver a result and a lot of personal struggle. Luckily, The Odyssey workout is geared to train you to get there a little bit faster and hard as it may seem, the personal struggle is nothing like its namesake.

Focus: Strength & Tone

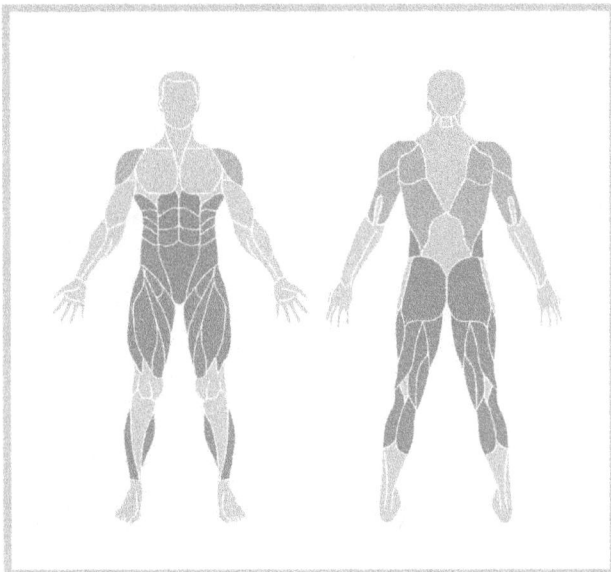

THE ODYSSEY

DAREBEE HIIT WORKOUT © darebee.com

Level I 3 sets **Level II** 5 sets **Level III** 7 sets | 2 minutes rest

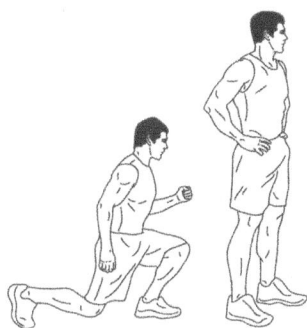

20sec reverse lunges

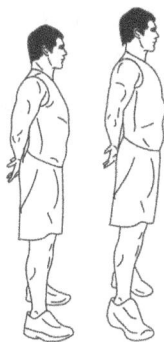

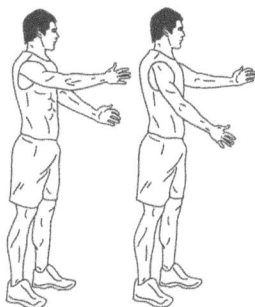

20sec calf raises

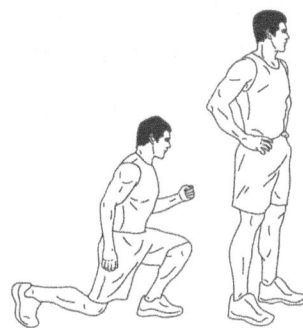

20sec reverse lunges

20sec scissor chops

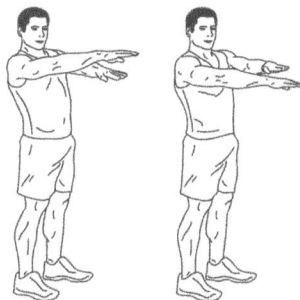

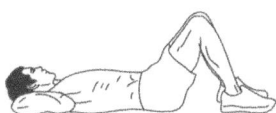

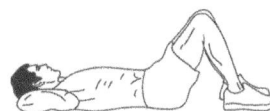

20sec arm scissors

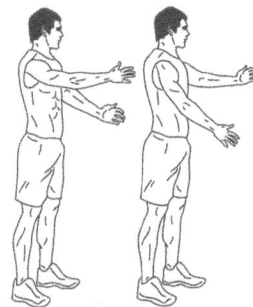

20sec scissor chops

20sec crunches

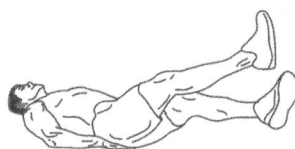

20sec scissors

20sec crunches

56 Off Day

On days when all you really want to do is stay in bed and watch Netflix you really need to get your body moving and your blood circulating. There are many reasons why you should, both mental and physical, but we won't go into them here. The Off Day workout is what you need. It's easy to do. It targets the whole body. It will not exhaust you. It will stop you from losing precious ground in your fitness and motivation.

Focus: Strength & Tone

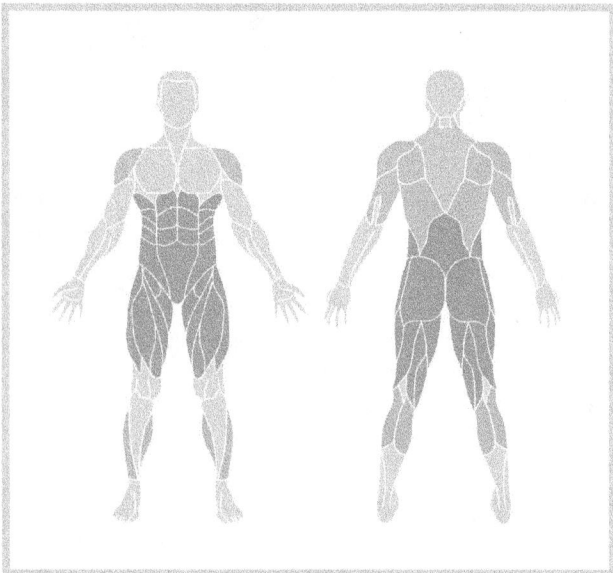

OFF DAY

DAREBEE WORKOUT © darebee.com

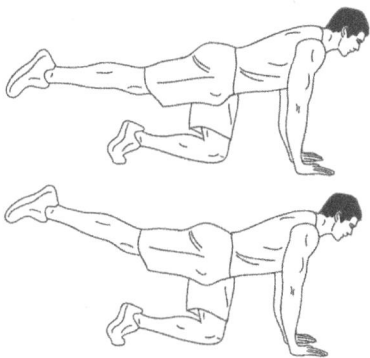

40 leg swings
switch sides and repeat

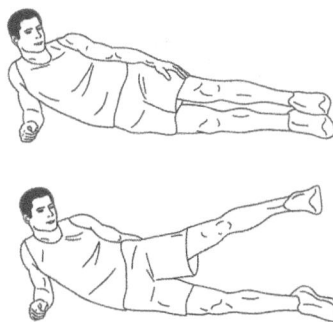

40 side leg raises
switch sides and repeat

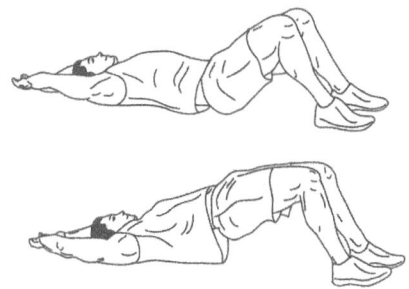

10 bridges x **4 sets**
30 seconds rest

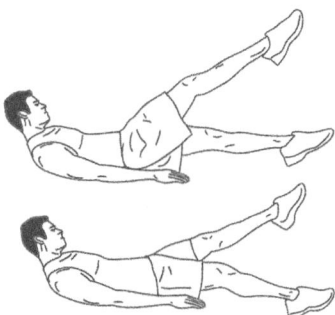

10 flutter kicks x **4 sets**
30 seconds rest

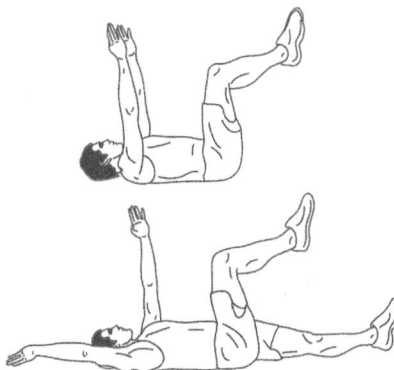

10 dead bugs x **4 sets**
30 seconds rest

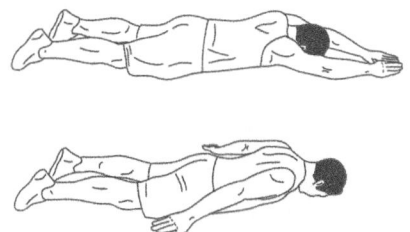

10 reverse angels x **4 sets**
30 seconds rest

57 One-Minute

One minute is all it takes to hit all the right muscle groups if the intensity of the workout is high enough. The One-Minute workout demands that you go flat out during each of the exercises, minimising down time as you transition from one to the next. While it may not be a truly hard workout it is, nonetheless one that will push all the right "get fitter" buttons.

Focus: High Burn

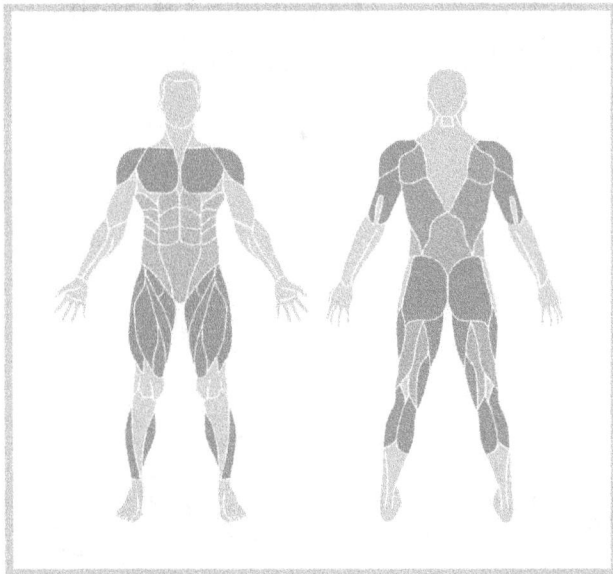

ONE-MINUTE WORKOUT

BY DAREBEE © darebee.com

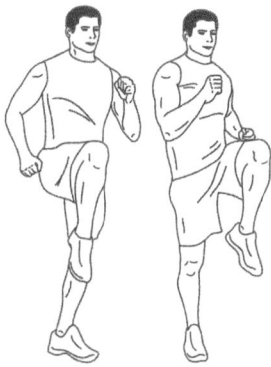

10sec high knees

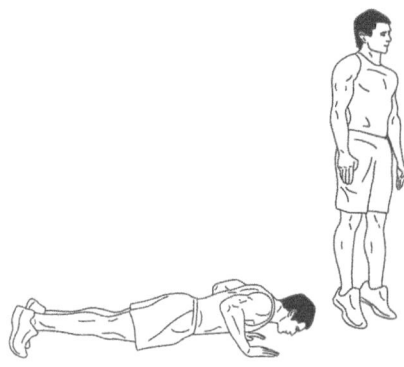

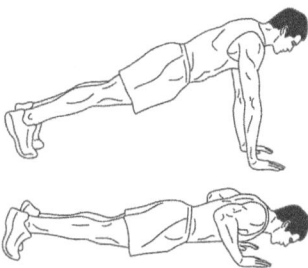

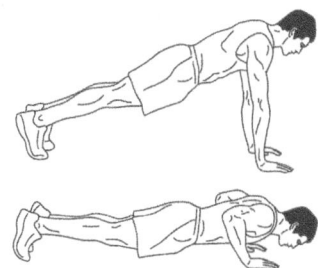

10sec burpees

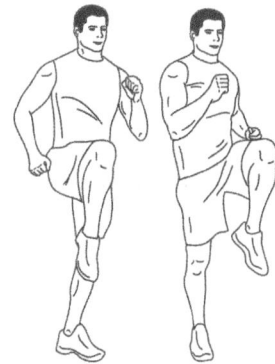

10sec high knees

10sec push-ups

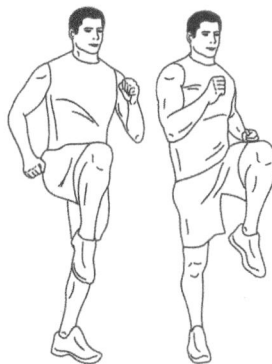

10sec high knees

10sec push-ups

58 Onna Bugeisha

Embrace your inner warrior and manifest your inner samurai with the Onna-Bugeisha Workout. This is a tough routine but so are you. This is your opportunity to be bold, be fearless, be - exceptional! Don't be afraid to put some power behind your kicks and punches as you go through the circuit.

Focus: Combat

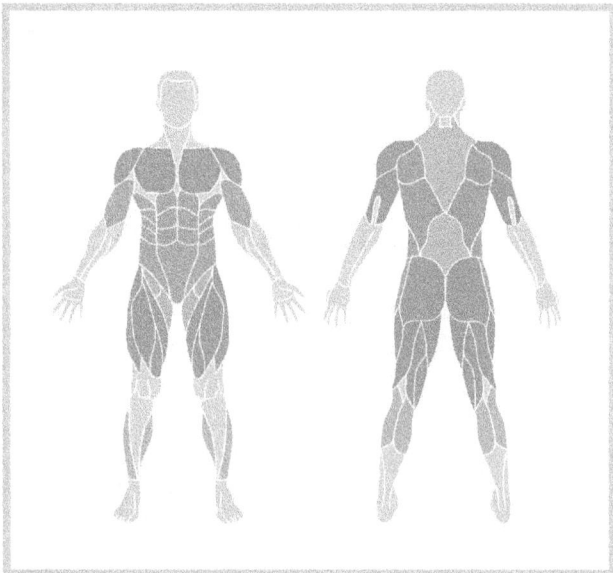

ONNA BUGEISHA

DAREBEE WORKOUT © darebee.com

LEVEL I 3 sets **LEVEL II** 5 sets **LEVEL III** 7 sets **REST** up to 2 minutes

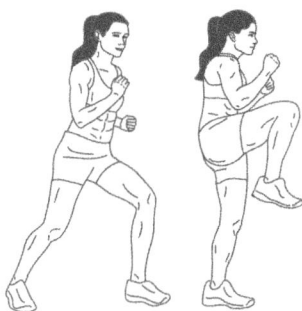

30 knee strikes

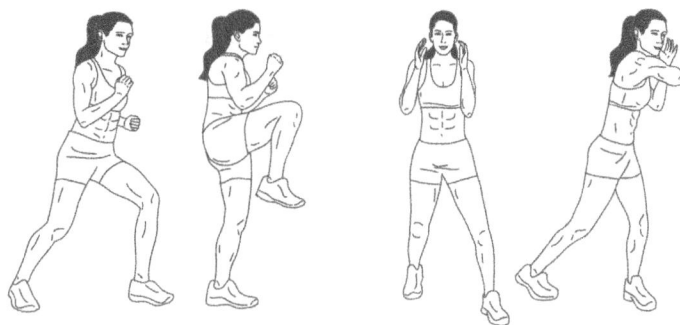

30combos knee strike + elbow strike

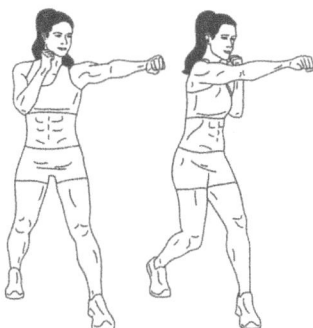

30 punches (jab + cross)

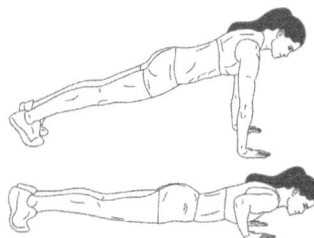

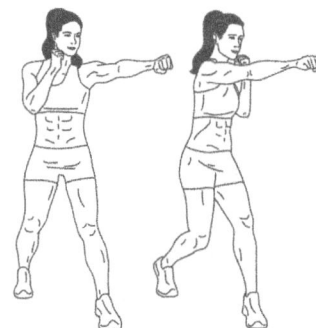

30combos push-up+ jab + cross

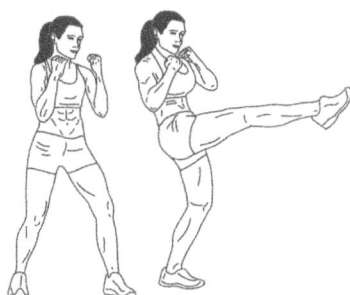

30 front kicks

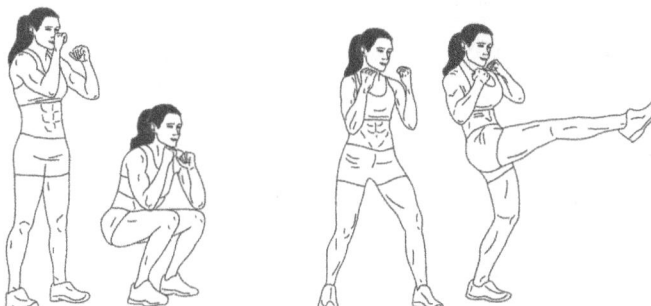

30combos squat + front kick

59 Outlaw

Outlaw is a combat moves, abs and core strength workout. It will make you sweat but it won't push you aerobically. It's not designed to. Go slow and steady in each move, pay attention to form and exercise muscles in their entire range of motion. The end result is a controlled, balanced workout that helps you maintain your edge.

Focus: Strength & Tone

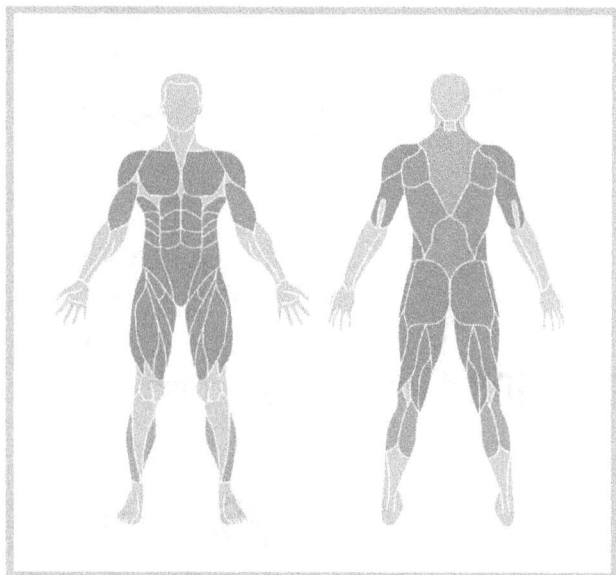

OUTLAW

LEVEL I 3 sets **LEVEL II** 5 sets **LEVEL III** 7 sets **REST** up to 2 minutes

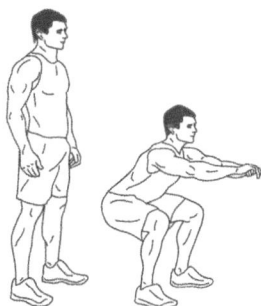

15 squats

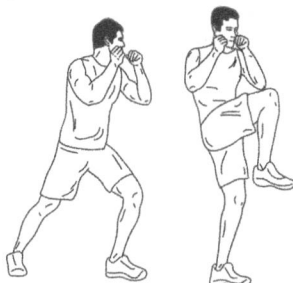

30 knee strikes

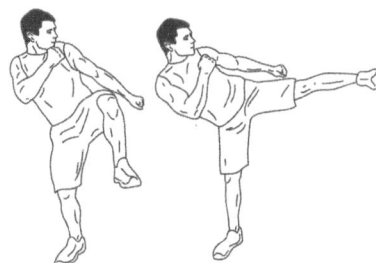

30 side kicks

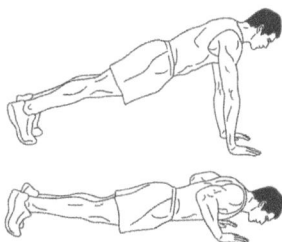

15 push-ups

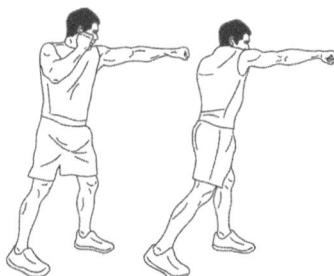

30 punches

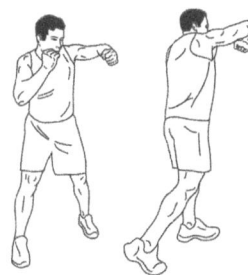

30 hooks

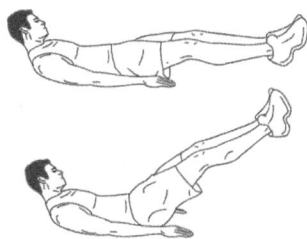

15 leg raises

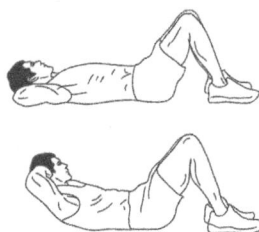

30 crunches

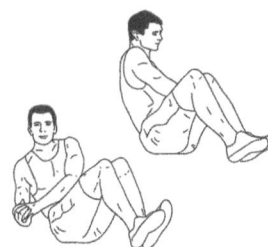

30 sitting twists

60 Overkill

Overkill is a high-load, fast-paced workout that needs you to minimize the transition downtime between exercises and make your body flow as you go from one to the next. This loads your muscles, lungs and cardiovascular system, gets you into the sweatzone fast and challenges your VO2 Max performance.

Focus: High Burn

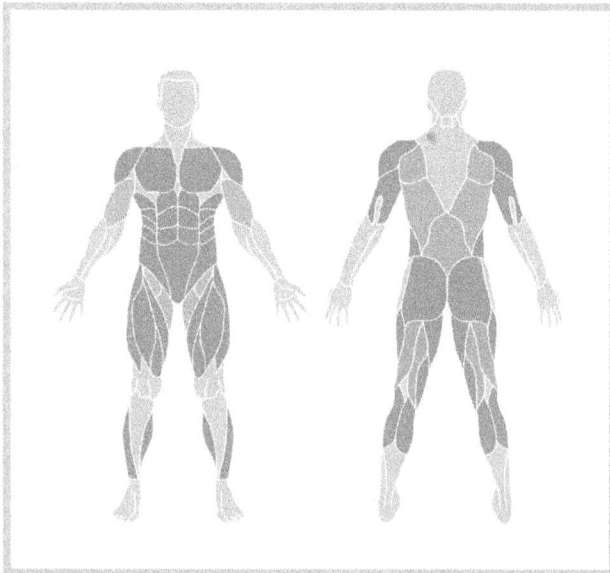

OVERKILL

DAREBEE WORKOUT © darebee.com

LEVEL I 3 sets **LEVEL II** 5 sets **LEVEL III** 7 sets **REST** up to 2 minutes

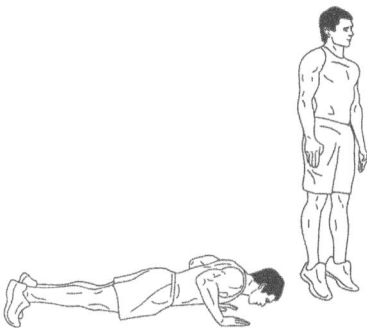

4 burpees

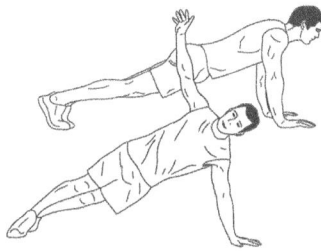

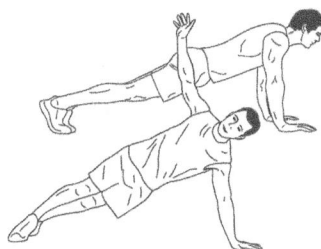

10 plank rotations

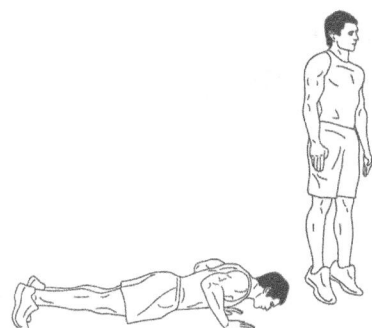

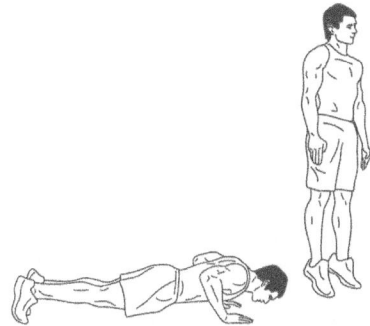

4 burpees

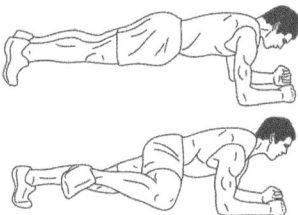

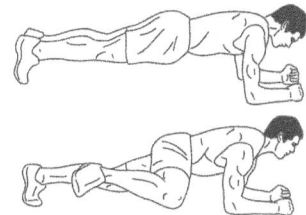

10 plank crunches

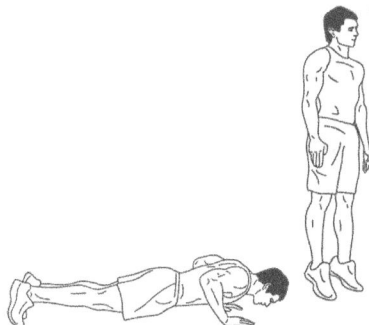

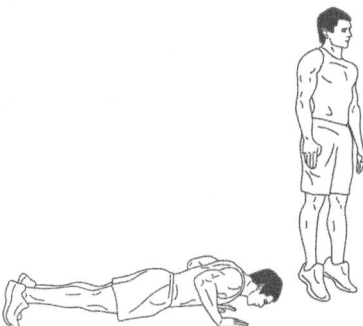

4 burpees

10 plank crunches

4 burpees

10 plank rotations

4 burpees

61 Over The Rainbow

Hyperload your muscles and then try to keep your balance! It's a lot harder than it looks. This workout is not just challenging (and extremely effective), it's also a lot of fun. Take a jump over the rainbow and see how you fair. You can change legs during balance hold halfway through or you can change sides at every set - it's up to you!

Focus: High Burn

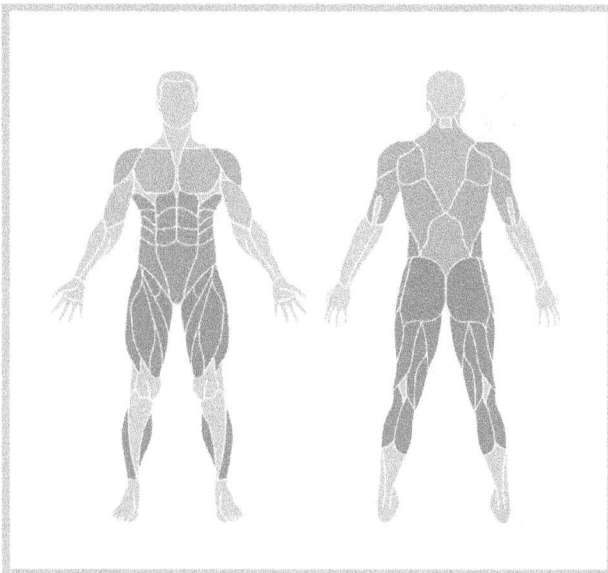

OVER the Rainbow

DAREBEE HIIT WORKOUT © darebee.com

Level I 3 sets **Level II** 5 sets **Level III** 7 sets | 2 minutes rest

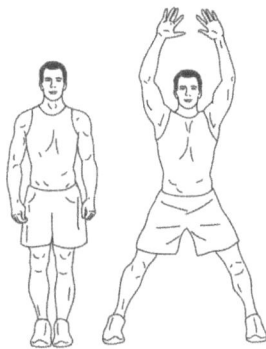

30sec jumping jacks

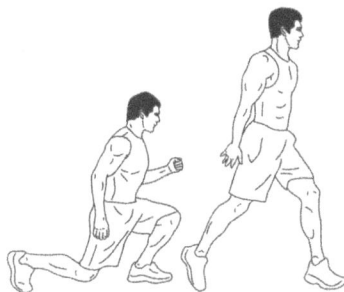

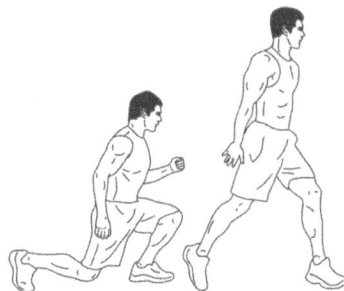

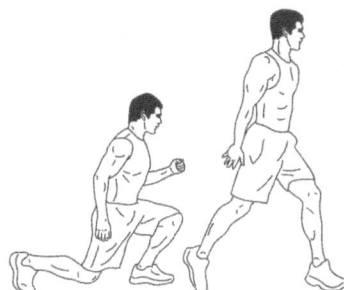

10sec jumping lunges

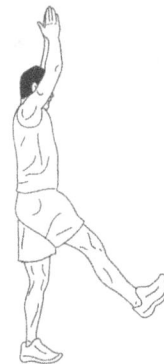

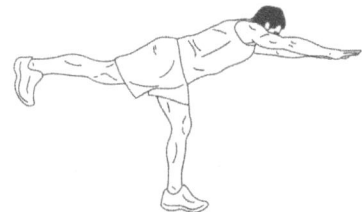

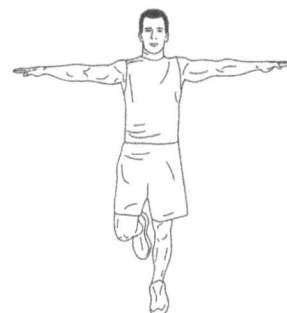

20sec balance hold #1

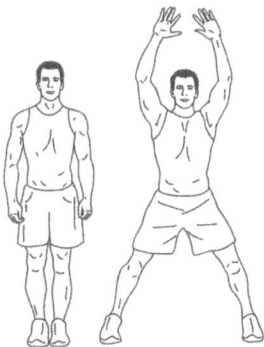

30sec jumping jacks

10sec jumping lunges

20sec balance hold #2

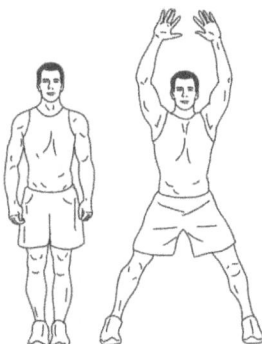

30sec jumping jacks

10sec jumping lunges

20sec balance hold #3

Pack A Punch

Compared to our size and weight our upper body is weak. This is why it takes the entire body to put power behind our punches. The Pack A Punch workout aims to address the imbalance by helping you develop the reflexive movements that repetitive exercise helps develop. Great for days when you don't have a lot of time to workout too.

Focus: Combat, Upperbody

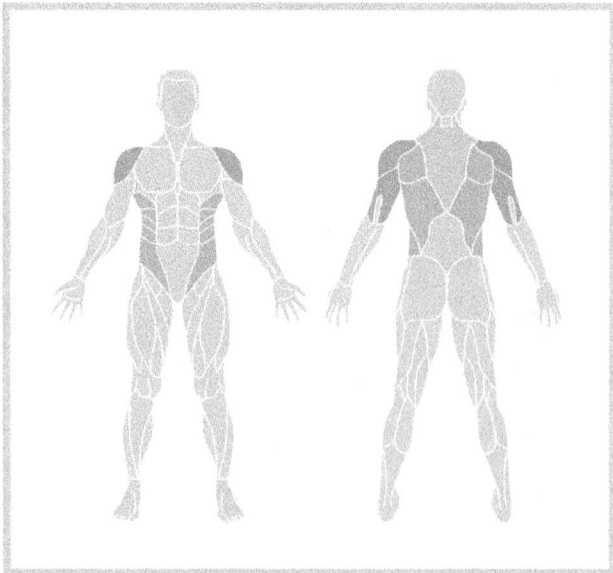

PACK A
PUNCH

DAREBEE HIIT WORKOUT © darebee.com

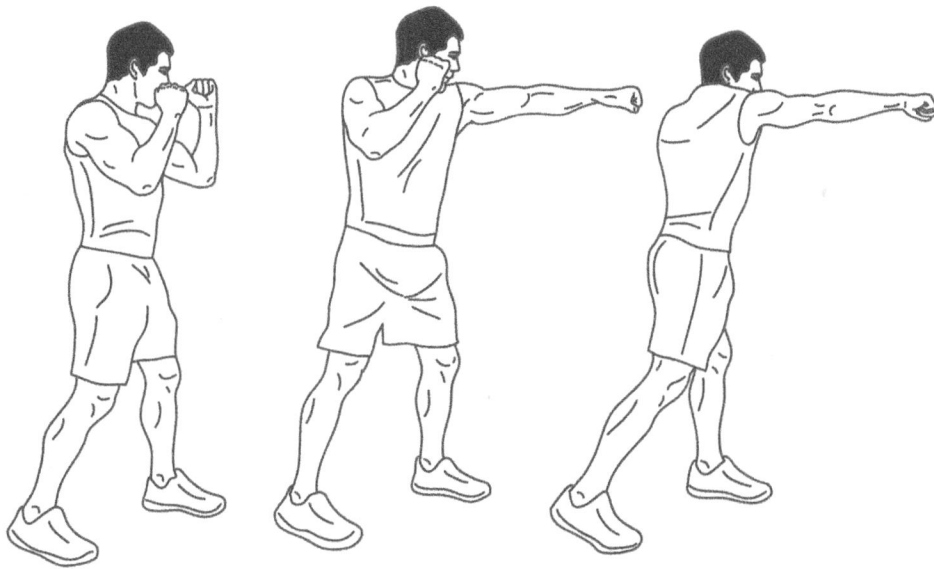

3min punches

30sec rest

3min punches

30sec rest

3min punches

done

63 Party Time

The Party Time Workout is perfect for recovery or as an active rest day routine. Get more out of it by picking up the pace and going through the circuit as fast as you can.

Focus: High Burn

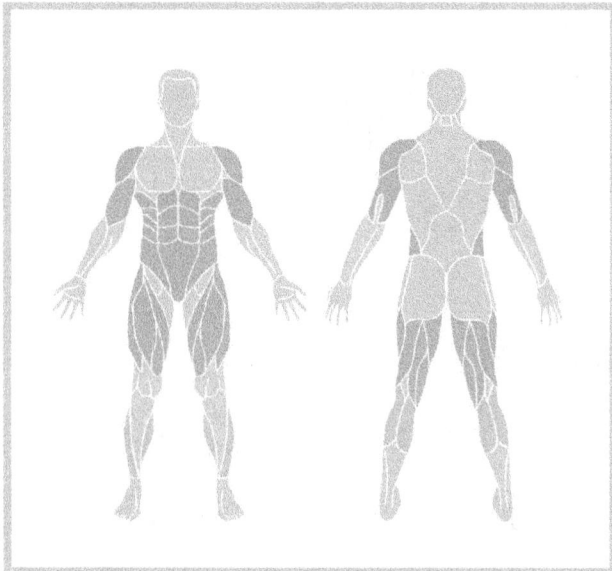

IT'S PARTY TIME

DAREBEE
WORKOUT
© darebee.com

LEVEL I 3 sets
LEVEL II 5 sets
LEVEL III 7 sets
REST up to 2 minutes

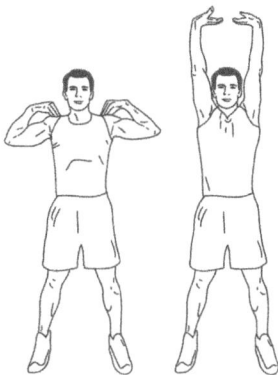

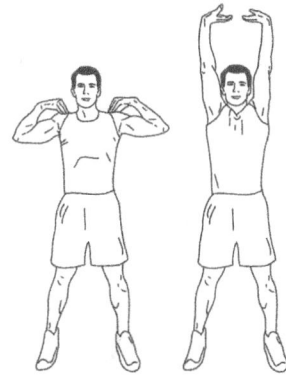

20 shoulder taps

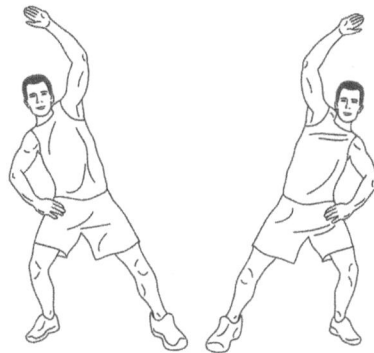

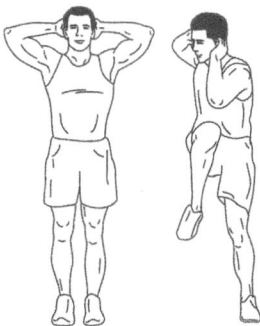

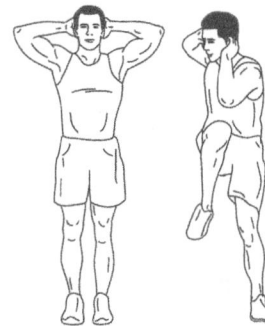

10 side jacks

20 shoulder taps

10 knee-to-elbows

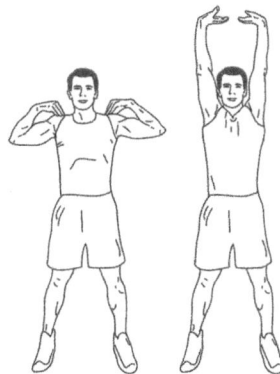

20 shoulder taps

10 knee-to-elbows

64 Permission Granted

The Permission Granted Workout is a full-body beginner-friendly routine for all fitness levels. It is a high burn workout with core and abs finish. During the circuit, focus on form rather than speed. Bring your knees to your waist when doing high knees and bring elbows in line with your shoulders when performing W-extensions.

Focus: High Burn

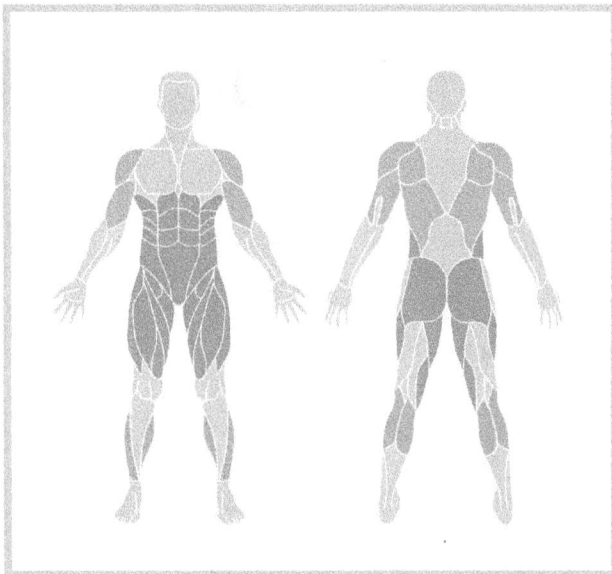

PERMISSION GRANTED

DAREBEE WORKOUT © darebee.com

Level I 3 sets **Level II** 5 sets **Level III** 7 sets | 2 minutes rest

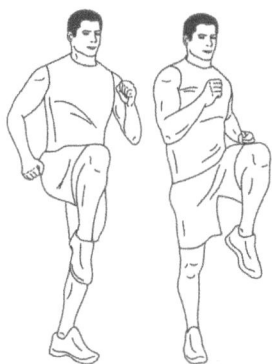

20 high knees

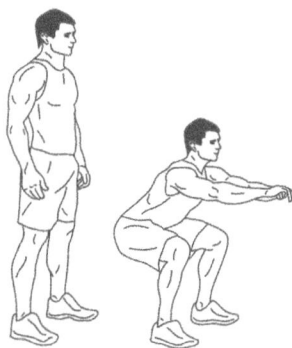

8 squats

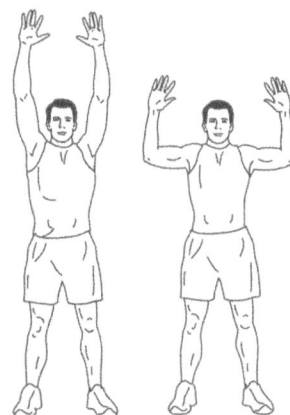

20 standing W-extensions

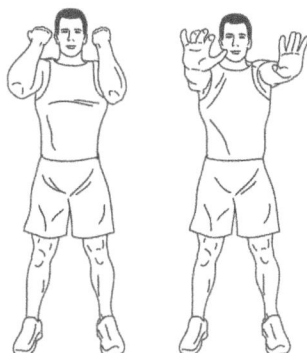

20 bicep extensions

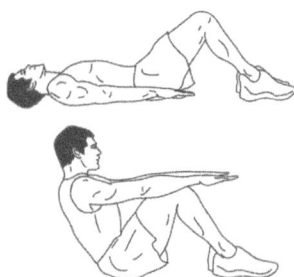

8 sit-ups

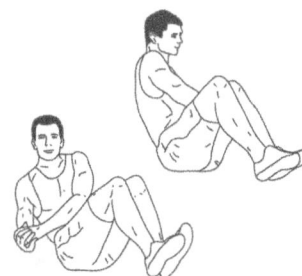

8 sitting twists

65 Player

When you have jump squats and push ups in one workout you just know you need to also add up and down planks as your downtime, core-training moment which means The Player is the workout to turn to. Especially designed to promote better fascial strength and fitness this is a workout that helps unleash the power of your body. Great for everyone doing contact sports, playing basketball or needing that total body explosion.

Focus: Strength & Tone

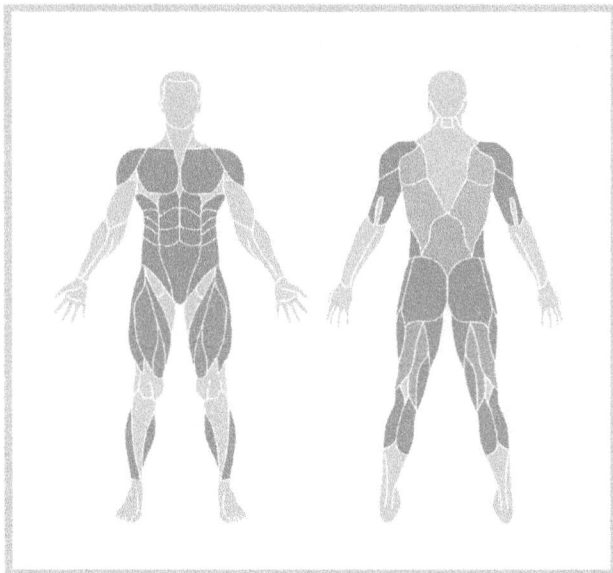

the Player

DAREBEE WORKOUT   © darebee.com

LEVEL I 3 sets **LEVEL II** 5 sets **LEVEL III** 7 sets **REST** up to 2 minutes

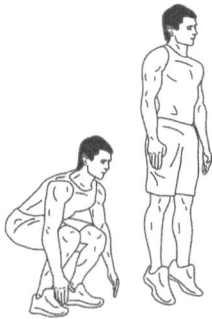

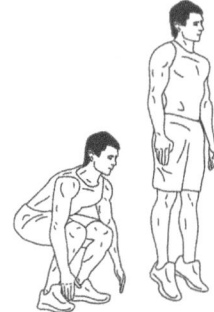

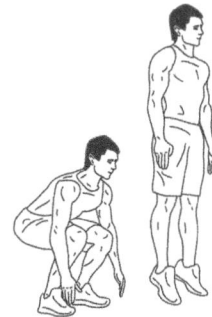

10 jump squats   **10** push-ups   **10** jump squats

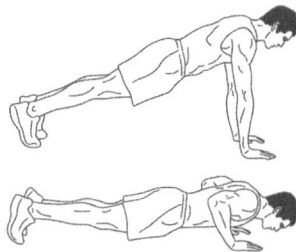

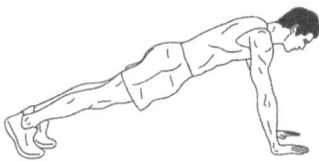

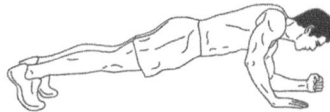

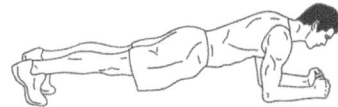

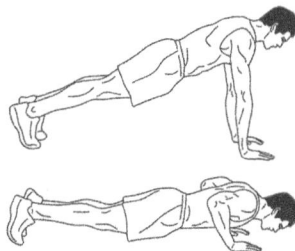

10 up and down planks

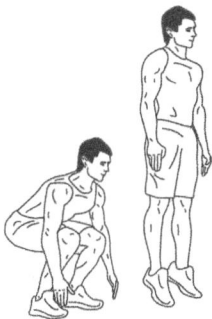

10 jump squats   **10** push-ups   **10** jump squats

66 Pouncer

The Pouncer workout will work your abs but it won't neglect the rest of your body. It looks deceptively easy and with just two alternating, time-based exercises you'd be tempted to think it is. The Pouncer has a bite however that begins to make itself felt after the first set. Treat with care. Come back to it often.

Focus: High Burn

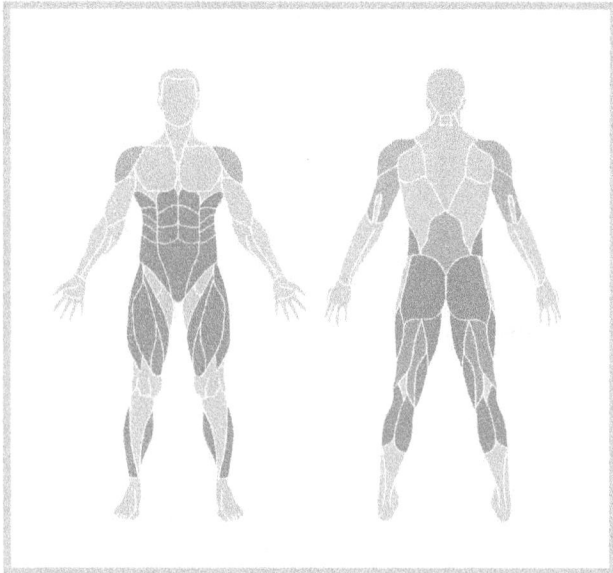

POUNCER

DAREBEE HIIT WORKOUT © darebee.com
Level I 3 sets **Level II** 5 sets **Level III** 7 sets
2 minutes rest between sets

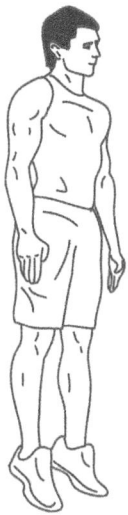

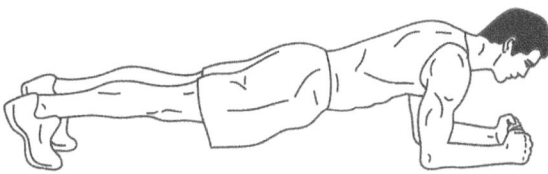

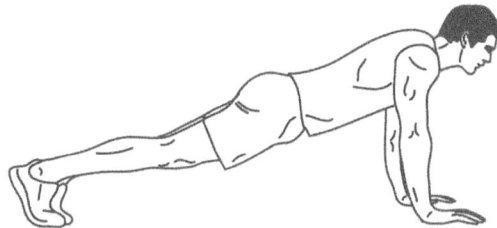

20sec elbow plank

10sec basic burpees

20sec elbow plank

10sec basic burpees

20sec elbow plank

10sec basic burpees

20sec elbow plank

10sec basic burpees

done

67 Powerbuilt

Powerbuilt may not look difficult but as a difficulty Level IV workout it is one that will let you know immediately that you've started to build up a load. Many muscle groups are recruited for each exercise making this a go-to choice for building up muscle strength. Pay attention to form and stay focused throughout. Your body will know the difference the day after.

Focus: Strength & Tone

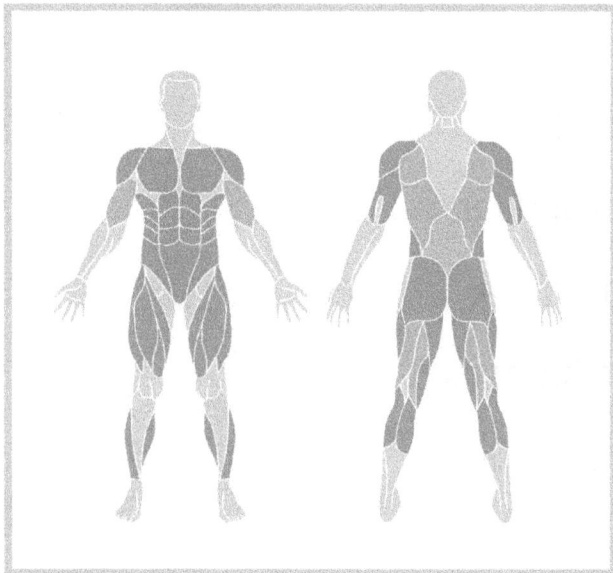

POWERBUILT

DAREBEE WORKOUT © darebee.com

LEVEL I 3 sets **LEVEL II** 5 sets **LEVEL III** 7 sets **REST** up to 2 minutes

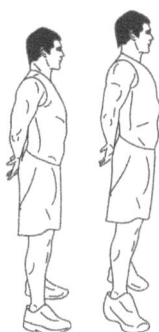

20 calf raises

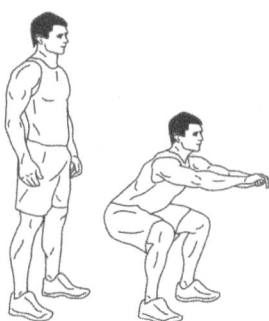

10 squats

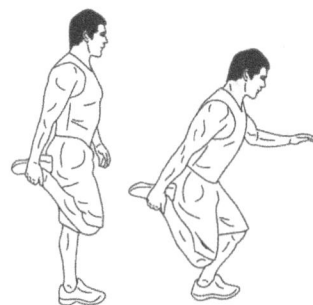

6 half shrimp squats

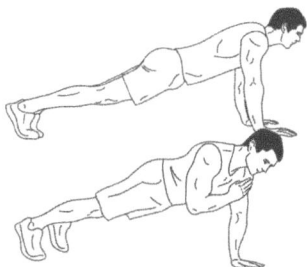

20 shoulder taps

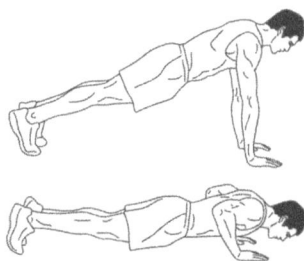

10 push-ups

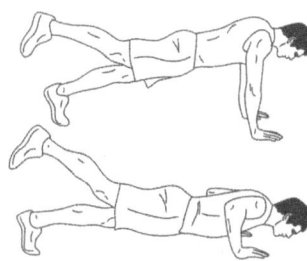

6 single leg push-ups

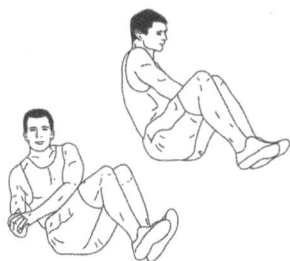

20 sitting twists

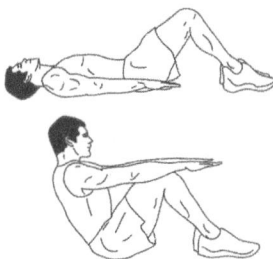

10 sit-ups

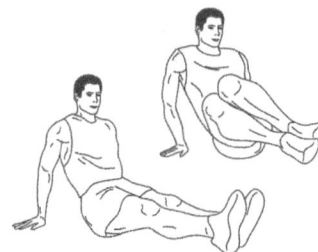

6 knee-in & twist

68 Power Burner

Power Burner is a Darebee workout that uses specific upper and lower body muscle groups and a little bit of impact to deliver a fascial fitness routine that helps with the body's natural elasticity and agility and helps build up explosive power. Its difficulty level is deceptive. Do it fast enough and with complete range of motion in each exercise and you have a fitness routine that will get you into the sweatzone fast.

Focus: High Burn

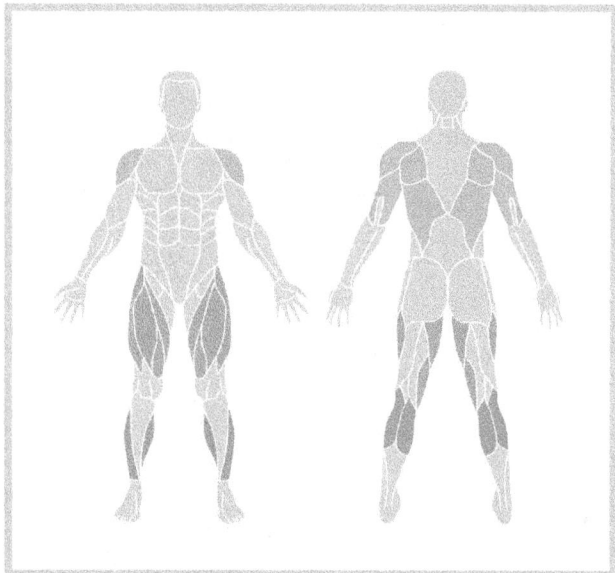

POWER
BURNER

DAREBEE WORKOUT © darebee.com
5 sets | 2 minutes rest between sets

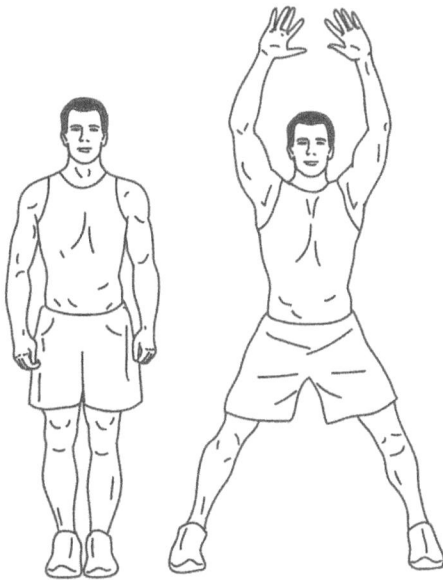

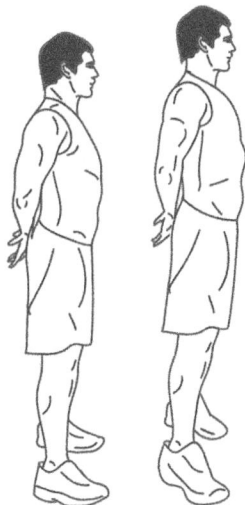

20 jumping jacks

5 calf raises

20 jumping jacks

5 calf raises

20 jumping jacks

5 calf raises

20 jumping jacks

5 calf raises

20 jumping jacks

5 calf raises

done

Power Gainer

Power Gainer delivers what it promises by strengthening major muscle groups in both upper and lower body, recruiting tendons and satellite muscle groups and increasing joint stability. This is a deceptive-looking workout that utilizes just four exercises to challenge the whole body.

Focus: Strength & Tone

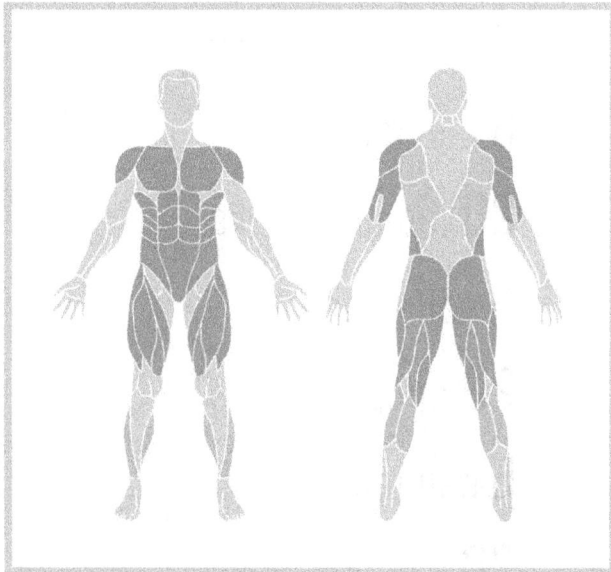

POWER GAINER

DAREBEE WORKOUT © darebee.com

2 minutes rest between exercises

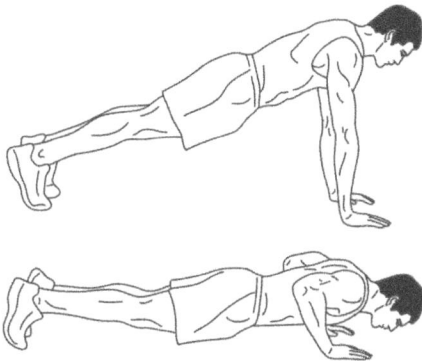

30 push-ups **x 3 sets** in total
30 seconds rest between sets

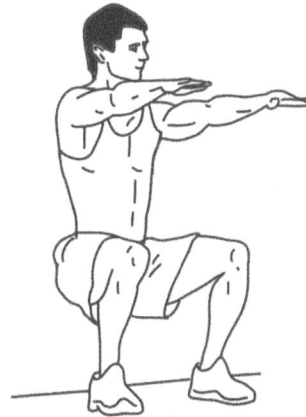

60sec wall-sit **x 3 sets** in total
30 seconds rest between sets

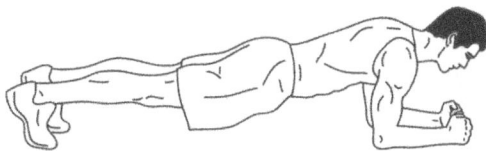

3 minutes elbow plank hold
once, in one go

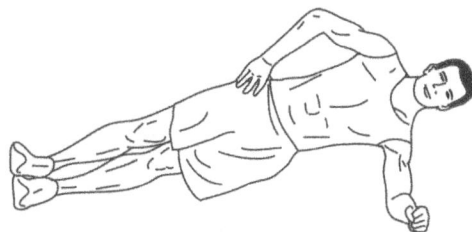

3 minutes side elbow plank hold
once, in one go

70 Pump & Burn

Pump & Burn is the workout you go to when you feel too tired to workout heavy. It's designed to be fast, light and energetic. It will keep you revving when you do not want to rev. Perfect for streamlining your body it has a strong aerobic component that will help you improve your endurance. Master it. You know you want to.

Focus: High Burn

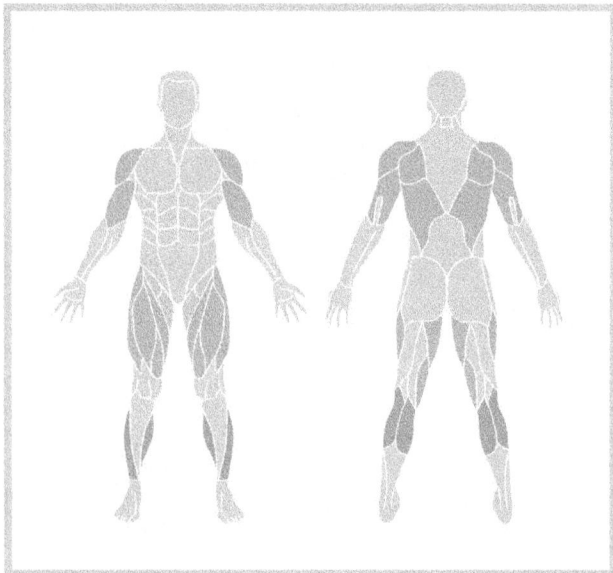

PUMP & BURN

DAREBEE WORKOUT © darebee.com

LEVEL I 3 sets **LEVEL II** 5 sets **LEVEL III** 7 sets **REST** up to 2 minutes

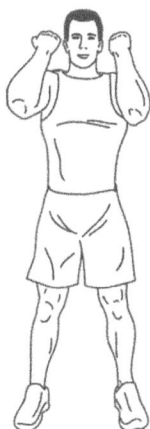

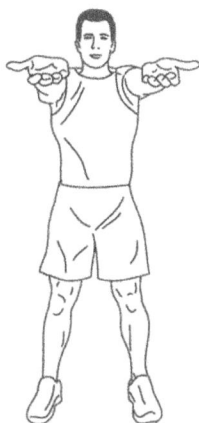

20 bicep extensions

10 jumping jacks

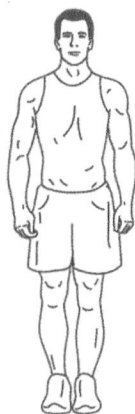

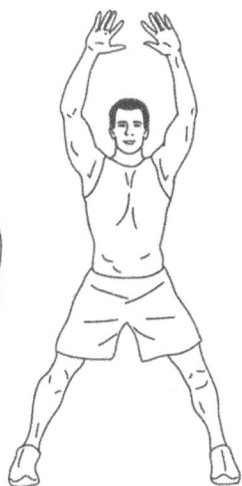

20 bicep extensions

10 jumping jacks

20 bicep extensions

10 jumping jacks

20 bicep extensions

10 jumping jacks

20 bicep extensions

10 jumping jacks

71 Quick HIIT

Sometimes you just need to HIIT it QUICK! Go flat out, de-stress, take over the world - you can do this! It has it all: cardio, combat, abs and core; all combined in one bad-ass workout. Keep your body straight while holding the plank. Don't drop your arms when transitioning from punches to squat hold punches.

Focus: High Knees

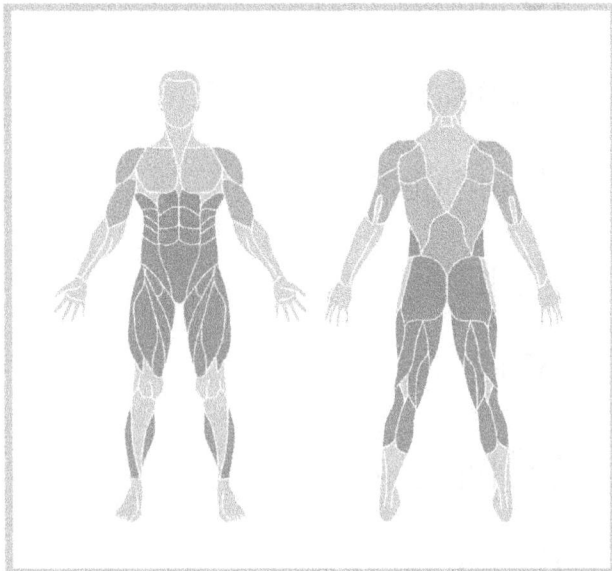

QUICK HIIT

WORKOUT
BY DAREBEE
© darebee.com

Level I 3 sets
Level II 5 sets
Level III 7 sets
2 minutes rest

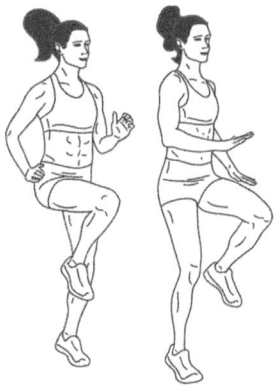

20sec high knees

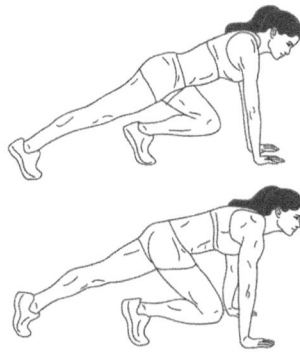

20sec climbers

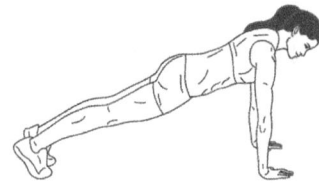

20sec plank hold

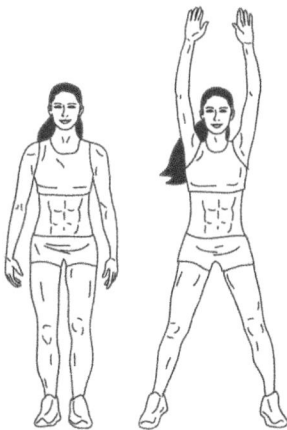

20sec jumping jacks

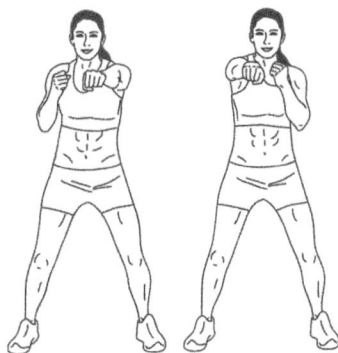

20sec punches

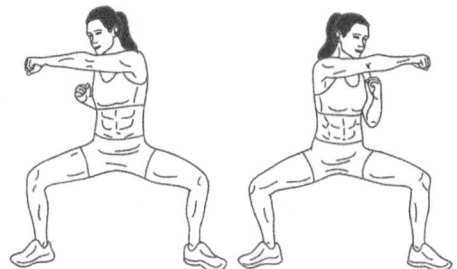

20sec squat hold punches

72 Rambler

Lower body work utilizes many muscle groups and requires a lot of coordination. It also burns significant amounts of oxygen to power all this. The Rambler is an HIIT workout designed to help you burn hot fast. Go for maximum rep count in each exercise in the allotted time and try to maintain the count throughout each set.

Focus: High Knees

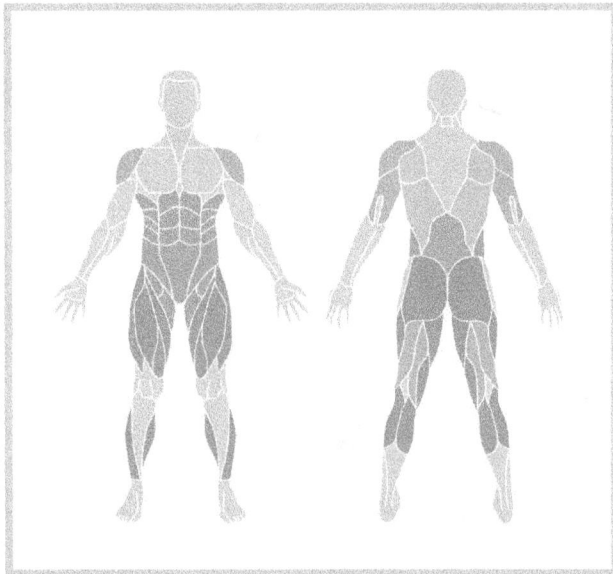

The Rambler

DAREBEE HIIT WORKOUT © darebee.com

Level I 3 sets **Level II** 5 sets **Level III** 7 sets | 2 minutes rest

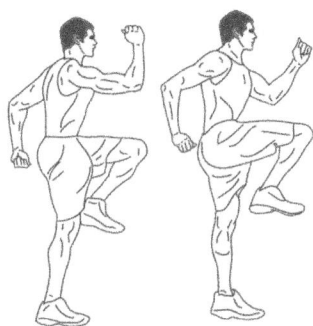

20sec march steps

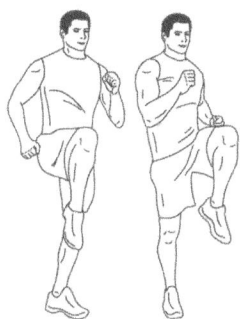

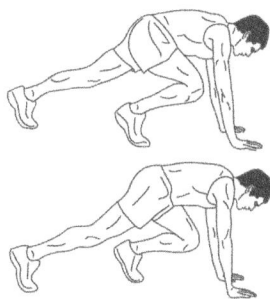

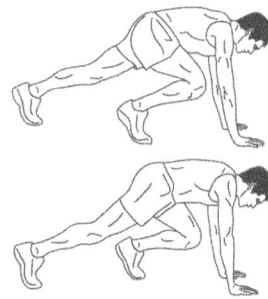

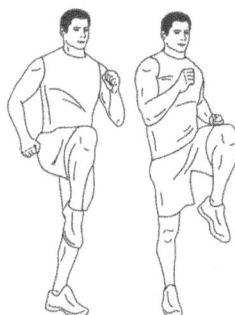

20sec high knees

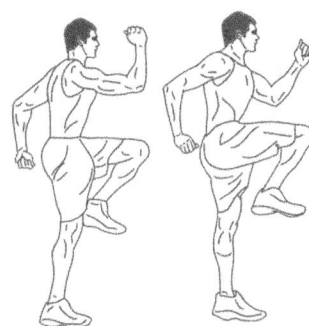

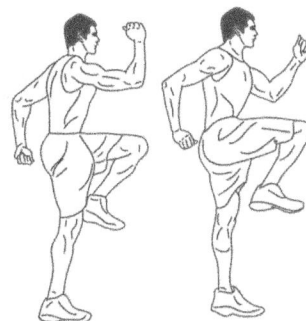

20sec march steps

20sec climbers

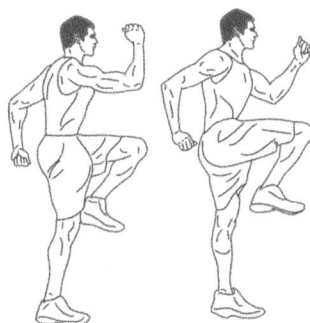

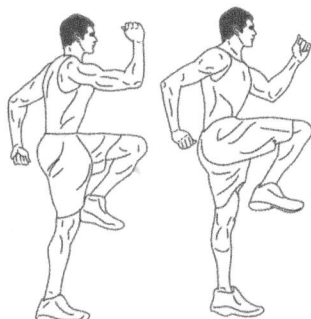

20sec march steps

20sec climbers

20sec march steps

20sec high knees

20sec march steps

73 Rascal

Rascal uses two exercises in alternating load mode to give you a fast, energizing, workout that delivers on effort and sweat but doesn't drain your energy banks. On a busy day when you might have to choose between a workout and staying fresh and sharp for that all-important meeting Rascal is just the thing you need.

Focus: High Burn

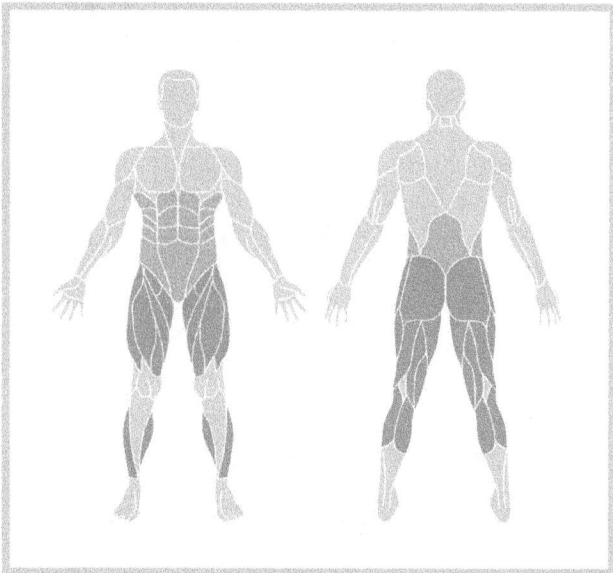

Rascal

DAREBEE WORKOUT © darebee.com
5 sets | 2 minutes rest between sets

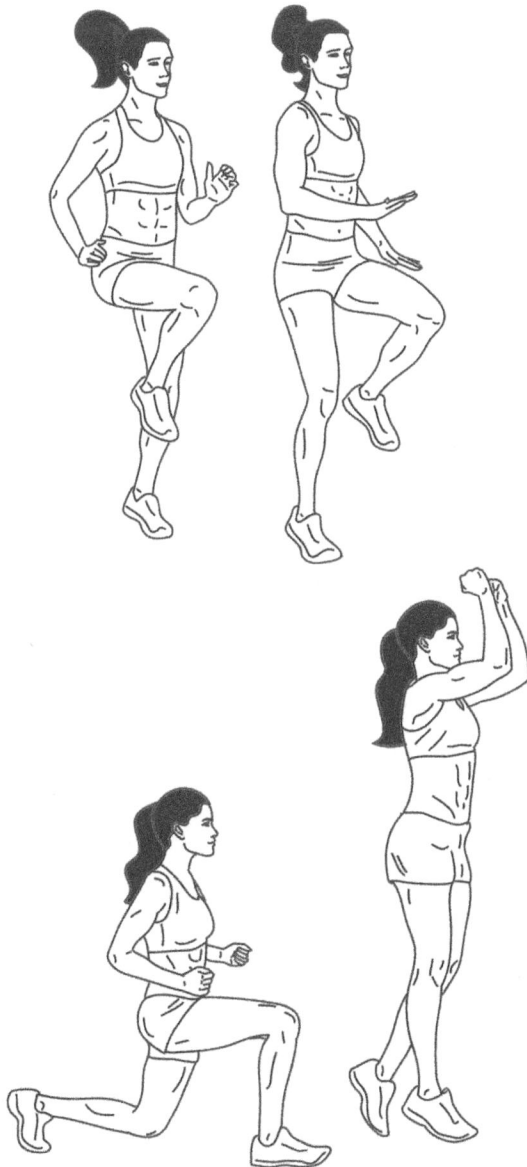

10 high knees

2 jumping lunges

10 high knees

2 jumping lunges

10 high knees

2 jumping lunges

10 high knees

2 jumping lunges

10 high knees

2 jumping lunges

done

Ravager

The Ravager is a workout that keeps on giving. Don't be fooled by it's simple structure and low rep count - it will make your muscles sing. Keep an even pace through the circuit and keep your head off the floor in the final ab work row for the best results.

Focus: Strength & Tone

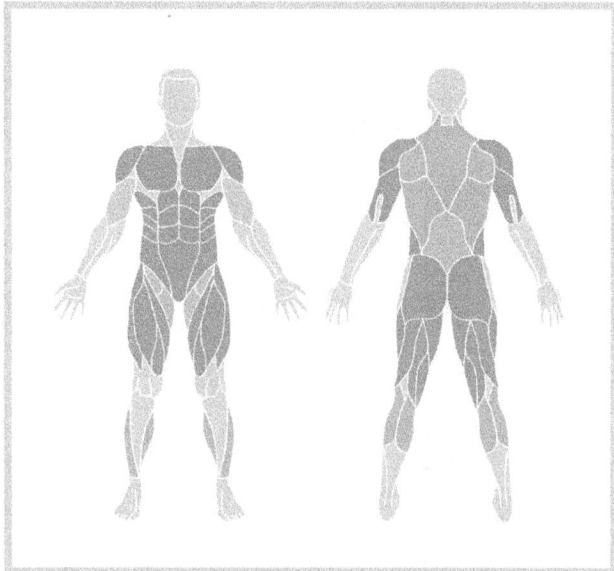

RAVAGER

DAREBEE WORKOUT © darebee.com

LEVEL I 3 sets **LEVEL II** 5 sets **LEVEL III** 7 sets **REST** up to 2 minutes

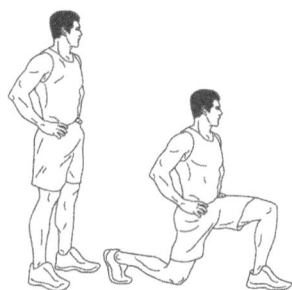

10 lunges

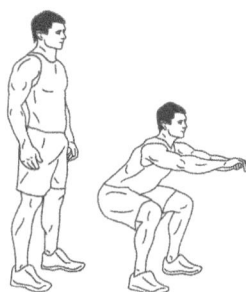

20 squats

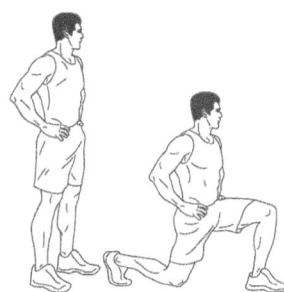

10 lunges

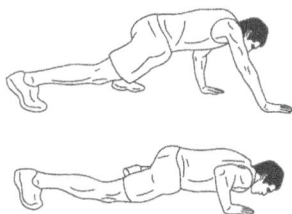

10 dragon push-ups

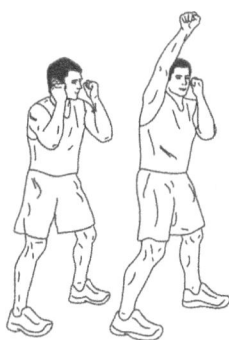

20 overhead punches

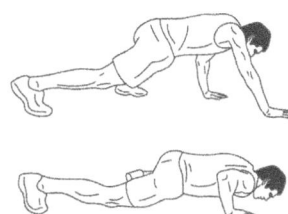

10 dragon push-ups

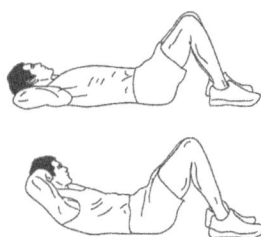

10 crunches

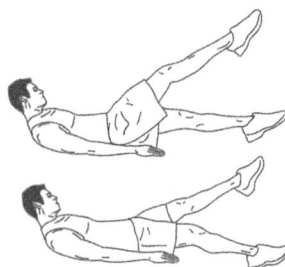

20 flutter kicks

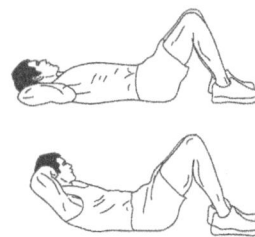

10 crunches

75 Raw Grit

Raw Grit will make you sweat, but it will not get you out of breath. This is a strength-building workout. Focus on technique. Make sure your form is as perfect as you can make it each time and maintain quality of execution throughout the workout.

Focus: Strength & Tone

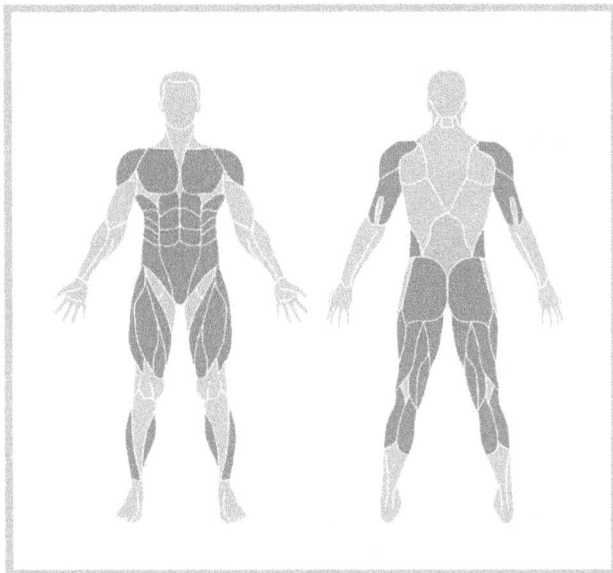

RAW GRIT

DAREBEE WORKOUT © darebee.com

LEVEL I 3 sets LEVEL II 5 sets LEVEL III 7 sets REST up to 2 minutes

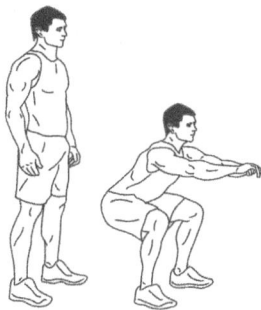

20 squats

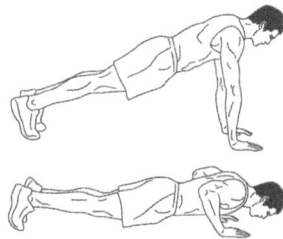

20 push-ups

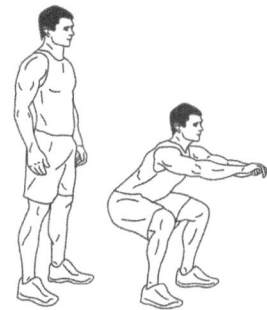

20 squats

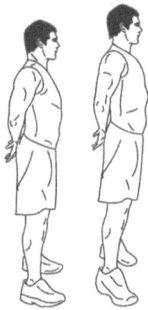

20 calf raises

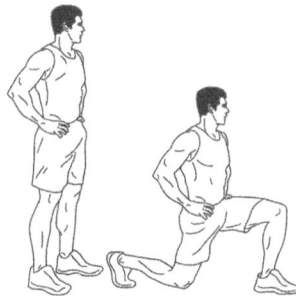

20 lunges

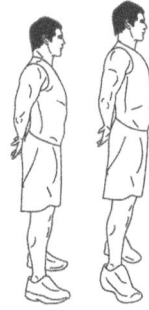

20 calf raises

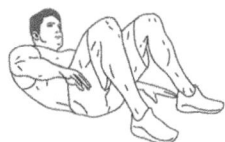

20 heel taps

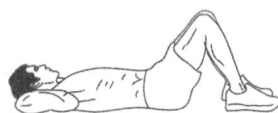

20 crunches

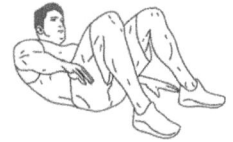

20 heel taps

Reconstructor

Remake your body, rebuild your muscles and find new strength. Well, after all that hype the Reconstructor workout had better deliver and yeah, that it does. Designed to load all your major muscle groups at almost the same time, it leaves you very little recovery time while you're exercising which means that you will definitely feel like you've worked hard with this one.

Focus: Strength & Tone

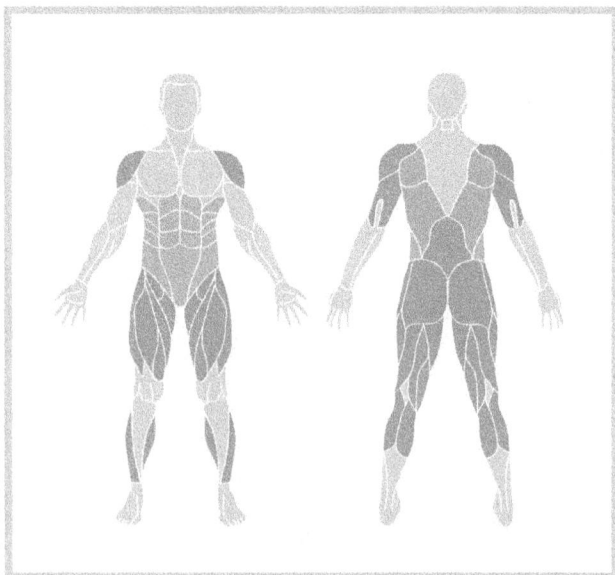

RECONSTRUCTOR

DAREBEE WORKOUT © darebee.com

LEVEL I 3 sets **LEVEL II** 5 sets **LEVEL III** 7 sets **REST** up to 2 minutes

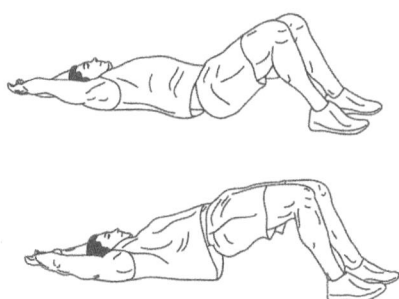

10 bridges

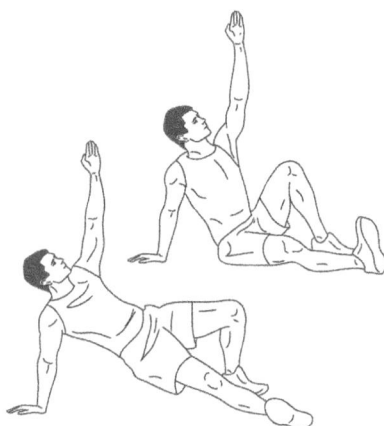

20 get-ups

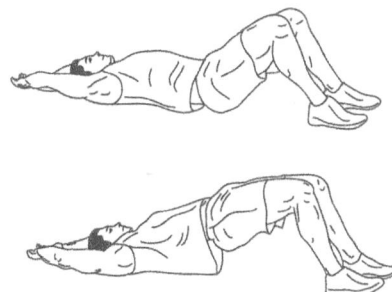

10 bridges

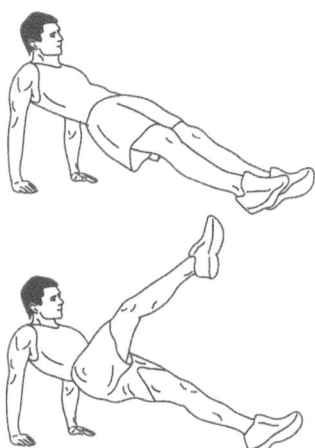

20 reverse plank kicks

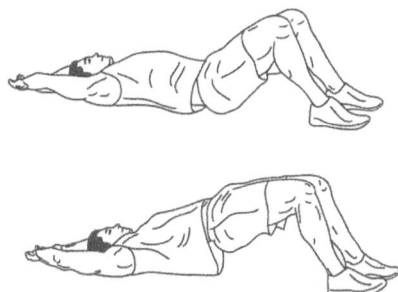

10 bridges

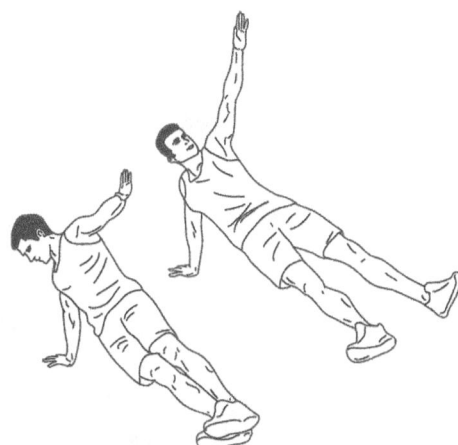

20 side plank tilts

77 Rectifier

HIIT exercises up your fitness level, improve VO2 Max and help you get fitter, faster. The Rectifier workout targets your whole body. Like every time-based workout reps and intensity are more important than form so you really want to try and get as many reps in for each exercise as you can and not drop your performance level as you go through the sets.

Focus: High Knees

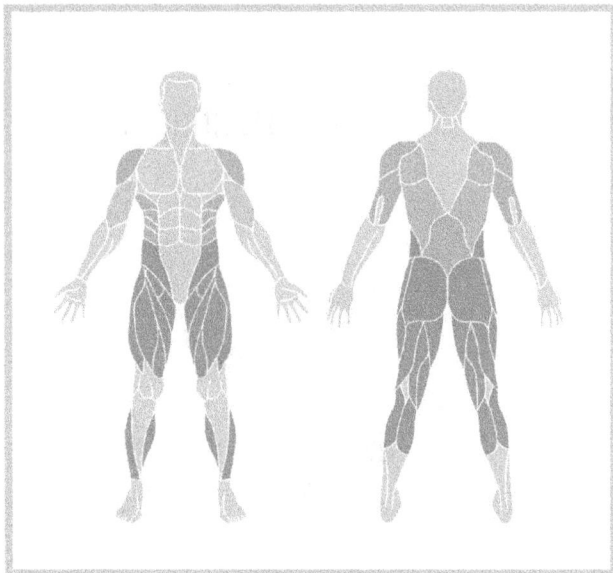

RECTIFIER

DAREBEE HIIT WORKOUT © darebee.com

Level I 3 sets Level II 5 sets Level III 7 sets | 2 minutes rest

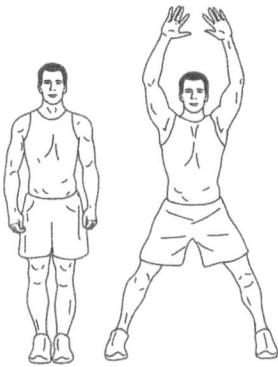

20sec jumping jacks

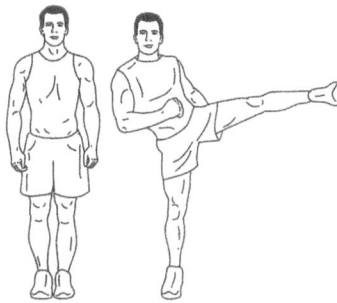

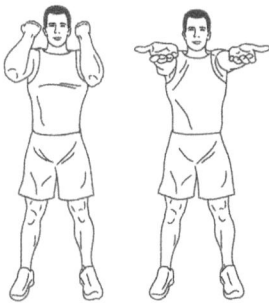

20sec side leg raises

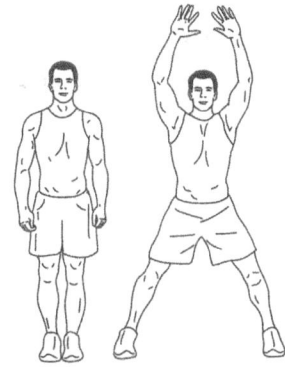

20sec jumping jacks

20sec bicep extensions

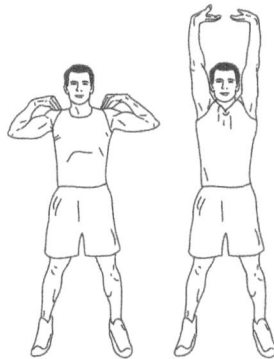

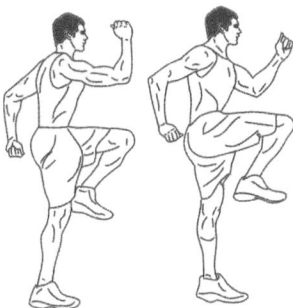

20sec standing shoulder taps

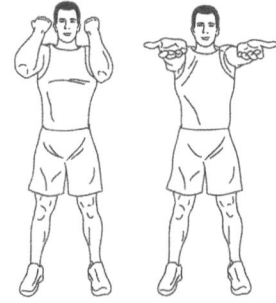

20sec bicep extensions

20sec march steps

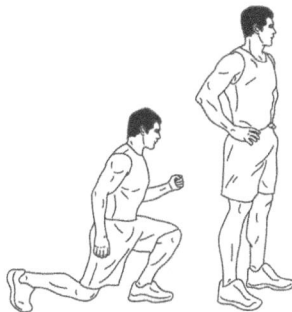

20sec reverse lunges

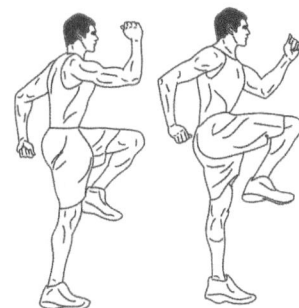

20sec march steps

78   Red Reaper

Chisel your upper-body strength and reinforce your core, become harder to kill with the Red Reaper Workout. Keep your body straight, tighten up your abs, take a deep breath - and dive in!

Focus: Upperbody Strength

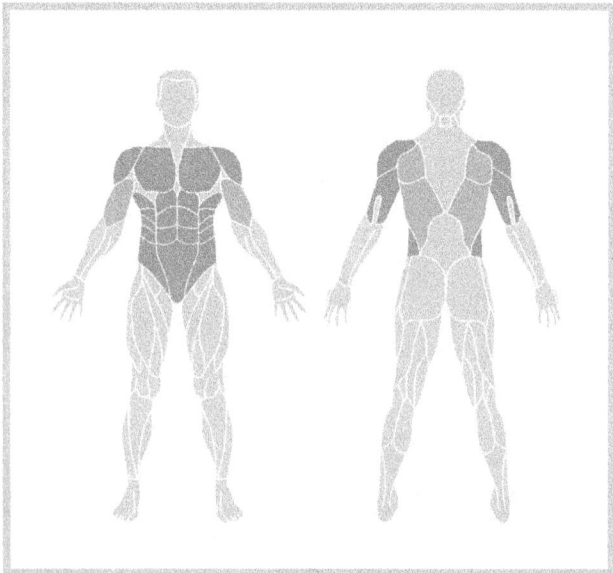

RED REAPER

DAREBEE WORKOUT © darebee.com

LEVEL I 3 sets **LEVEL II** 5 sets **LEVEL III** 7 sets **REST** up to 2 minutes

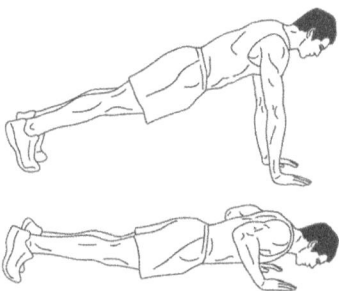

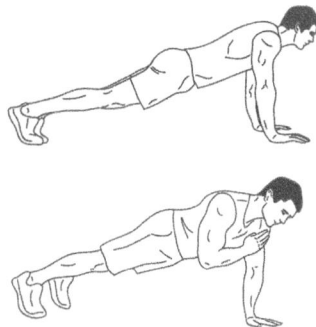

15 push-ups   **30** shoulder taps   **15** push-ups

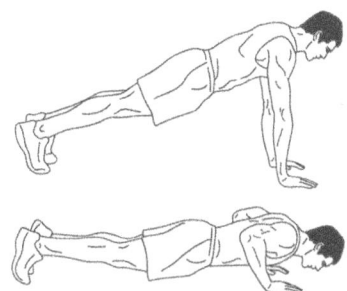

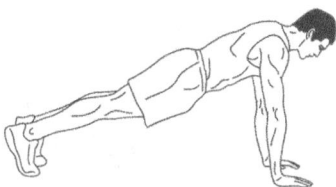

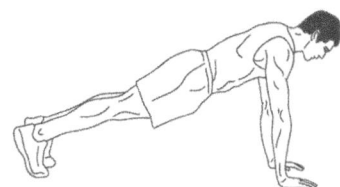

15-count plank hold   **30** plank side crunches   **15-count** plank hold

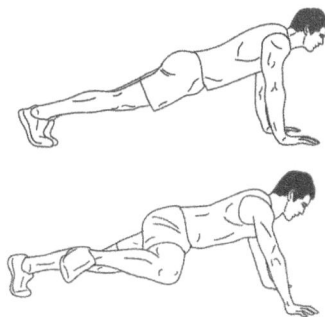

Rest & Rec

Res & Rec is a deceptively named workout, at least as far as the first part of its name is concerned. The exercises target tendons and support muscle groups that are not normally targeted during regular workouts. As such it helps to build up a good sense of body control. Do not neglect to add this workout to the arsenal of body modification ones you have already. (You do have a list, right?).

Focus: Wellbeing

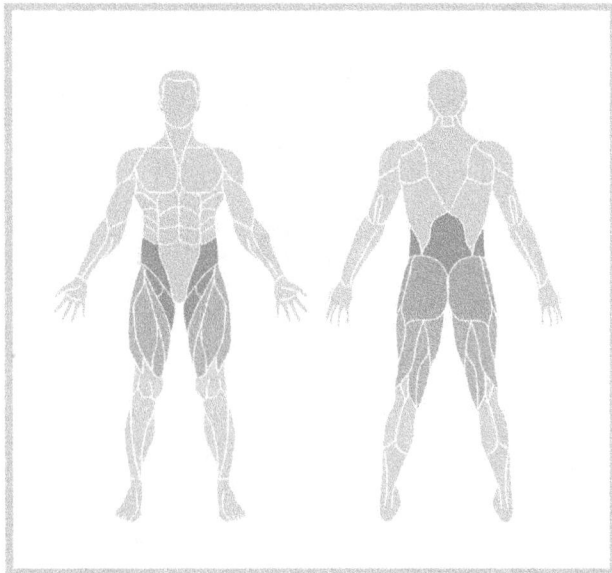

REST & REC

DAREBEE
RECOVERY
WORKOUT
© darebee.com

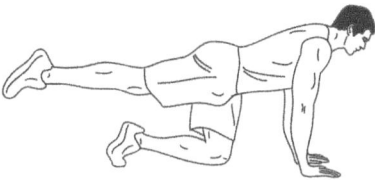
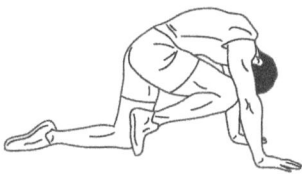

40 knee-ins

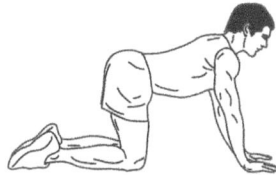
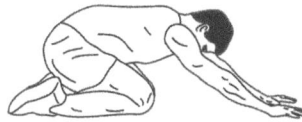

10 back stretch #1

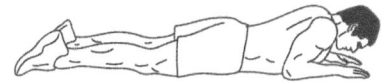
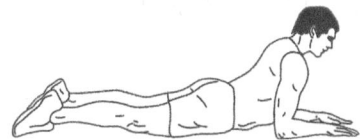

10 back stretch #2

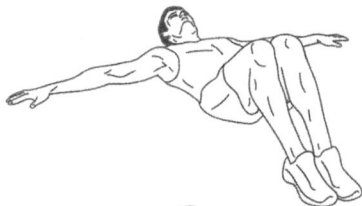

40 knee rolls

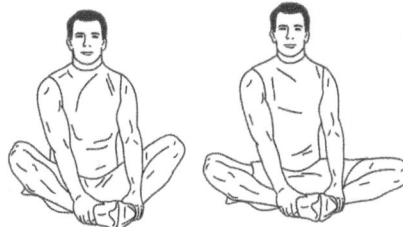

10 butterfly stretch

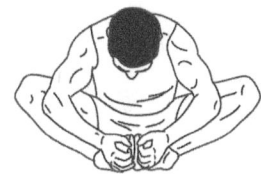

10 forward fold

80	Reviver

Get back on track with the Reviver Workout. It's an accessible HIIT workout ideal for when you are sore or in recovery but still need an exercise fix. Keep your arms up during bicep extensions and tighten up your core during planks.

Focus: High Knees

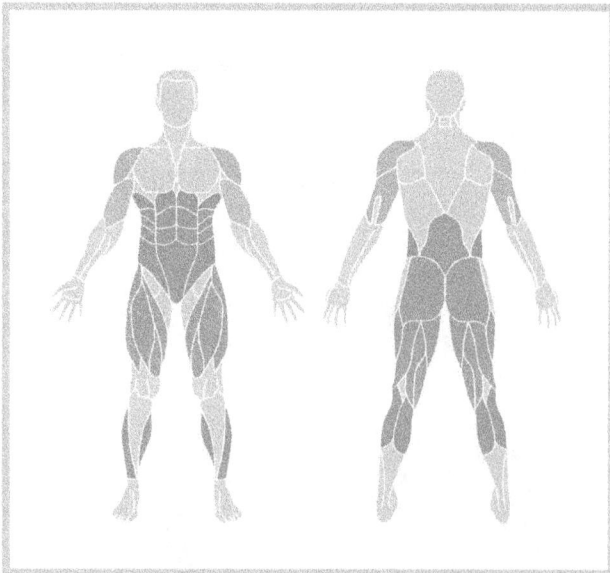

REVIVER

DAREBEE HIIT WORKOUT © darebee.com

Level I 3 sets Level II 5 sets Level III 7 sets | 2 minutes rest

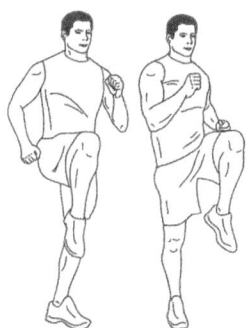

30sec high knees

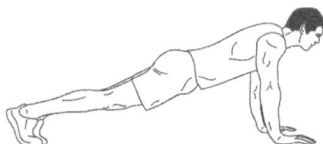

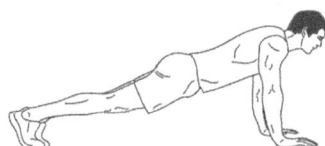

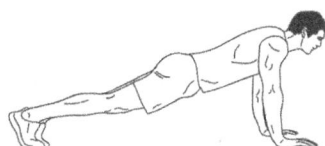

20sec plank hold

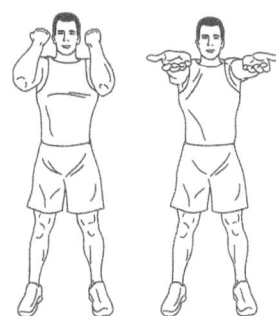

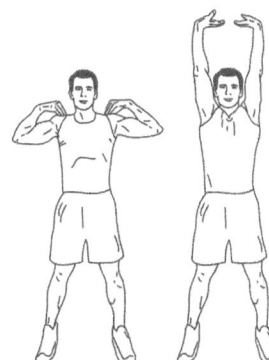

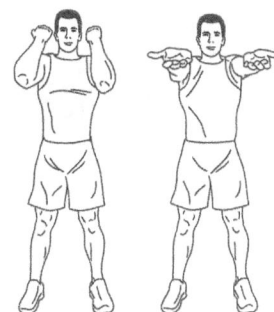

10sec bicep extensions

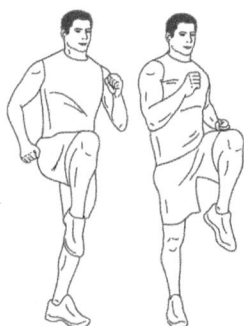

30sec high knees

20sec plank hold

10sec shoulder taps

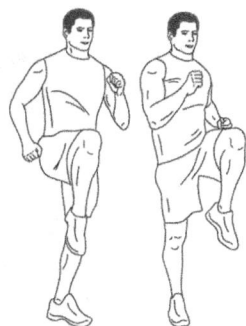

30sec high knees

20sec plank hold

10sec bicep extensions

81 Rewired

The Rewired Workout is hard enough to get you working but not too demanding to make you regret it. If you feel it's time to shake off the cobwebs and give your system a full defrag - this is the workout for you. Keep your body straight during planks and go full out during jumping jacks.

Focus: High Knees

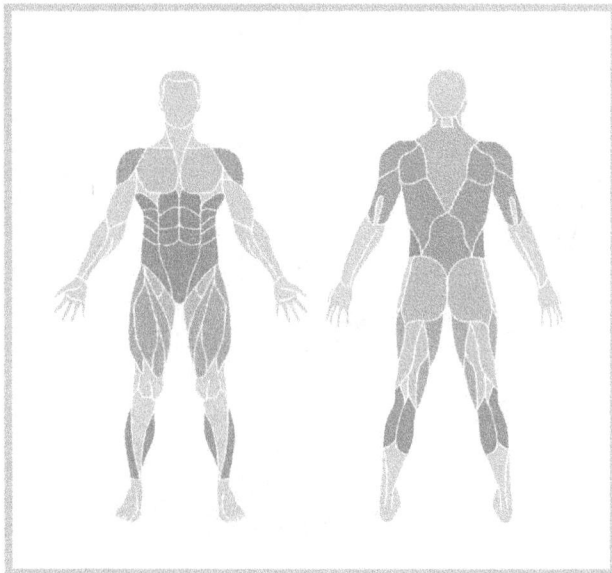

REWIRED

DAREBEE `HIIT` WORKOUT © darebee.com

Level I 3 sets **Level II** 5 sets **Level III** 7 sets | 2 minutes rest

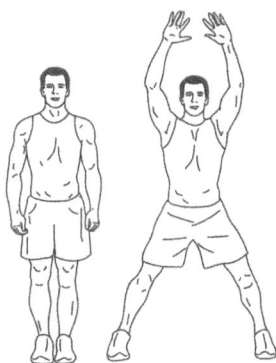

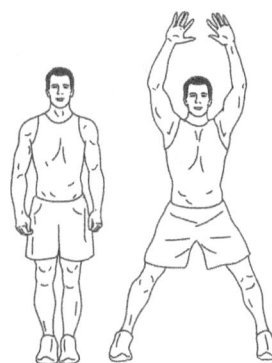

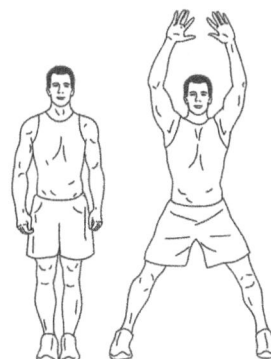

20sec jumping jacks   **20sec** plank rotations   **20sec** jumping jacks

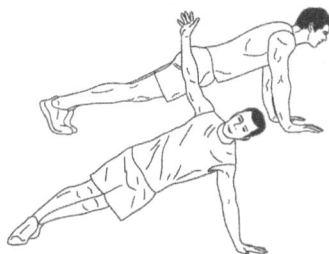

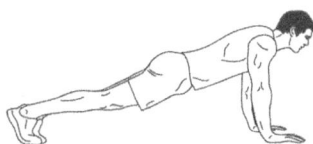

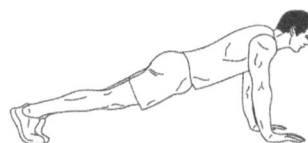

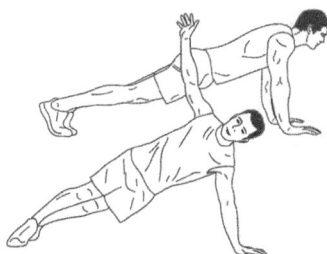

20sec plank hold   **20sec** jumping jacks   **20sec** plank hold

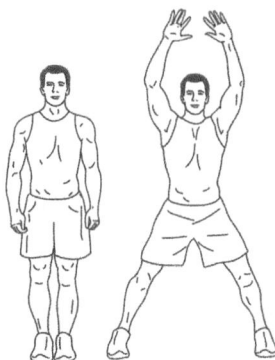

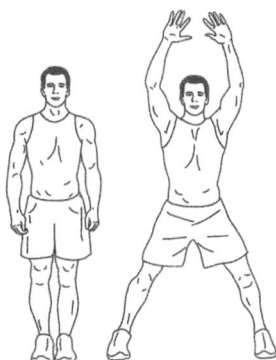

20sec jumping jacks   **20sec** plank rotations   **20sec** jumping jacks

82 Ricochet

Combat moves when coupled with callisthenics produce an interesting challenge: muscles have to work ballistically and with resistance which means the dynamic range of motion is challenged both ways. Ricochet provides a workout that will tire you out faster than you expect and will challenge your conditioning. Then again that's what you're here for.

Focus: High Knees

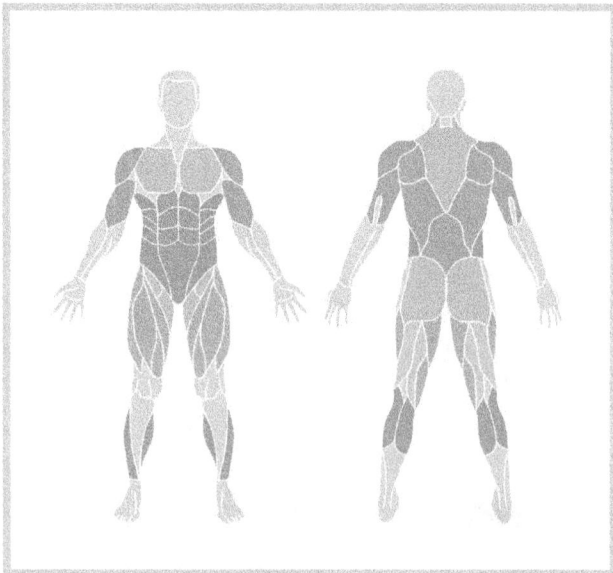

RICOCHET

DAREBEE HIIT WORKOUT © darebee.com

Level I 3 sets **Level II** 5 sets **Level III** 7 sets

2 minutes rest between set

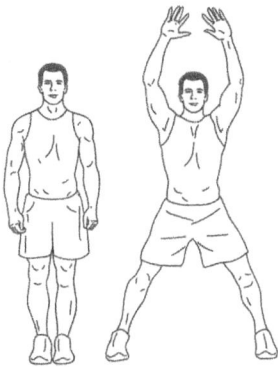

30sec jumping jacks

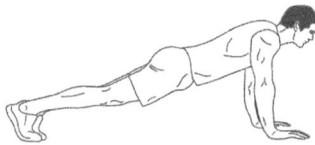

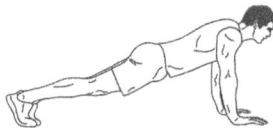

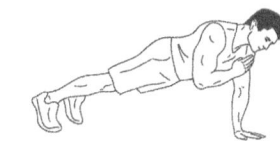

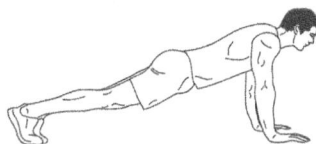

15sec plank hold

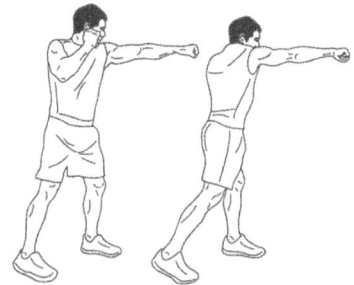

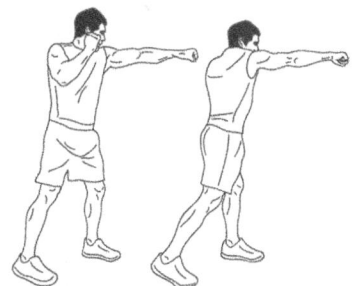

15sec punches

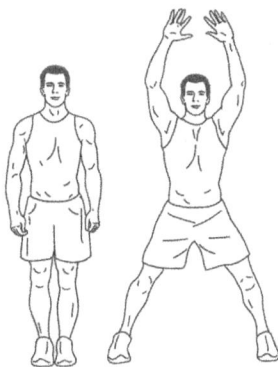

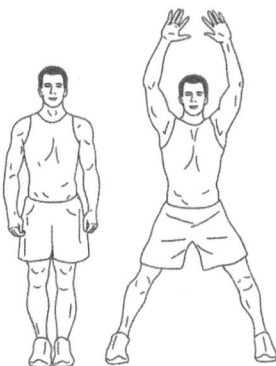

30sec jumping jacks

15sec shoulder taps

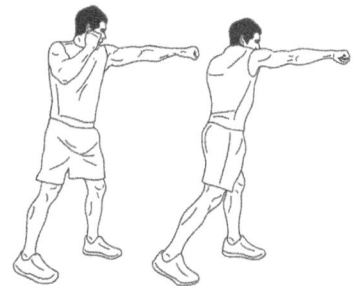

15sec punches

30sec jumping jacks

15sec plank hold

15sec punches

83 Rockin' Abs

Rockin' Hard Abs don't just happen. This routine will help you get closer to the abs of steel! And it will also work those glutes in the process. Go slow and focus on form. When performing leg raises lower your feet almost all the way to the floor but don't drop them, then raise them back up again.

Focus: Abs

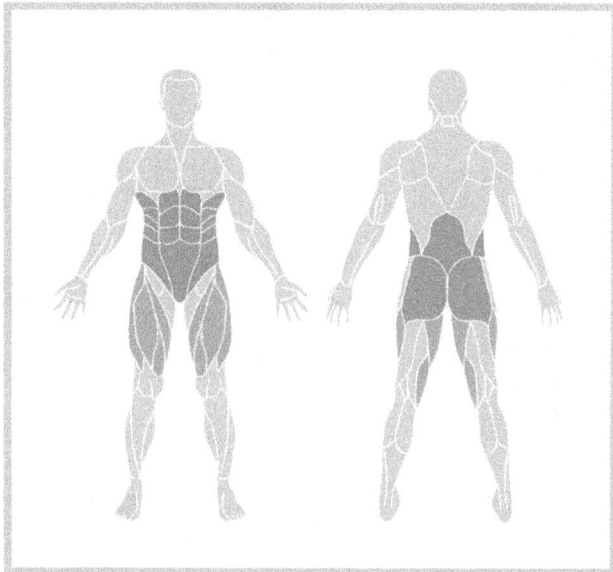

rockin' abs

DAREBEE WORKOUT © darebee.com

LEVEL I 3 sets **LEVEL II** 4 sets **LEVEL III** 5 sets **REST** up to 2 minutes

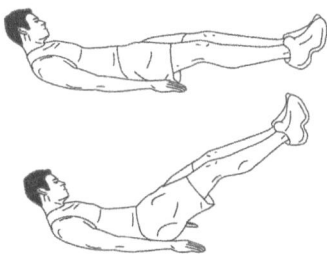

10 leg raises

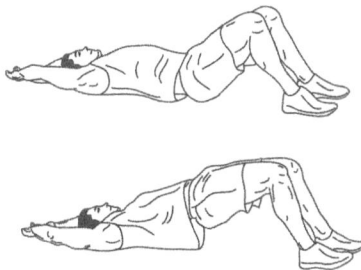

5 bridges

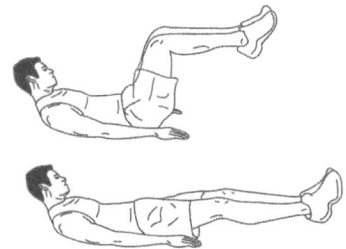

10 crunch kicks

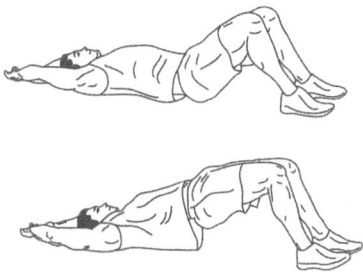

5 bridges

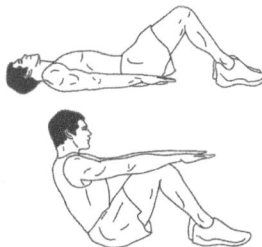

10 sit-ups

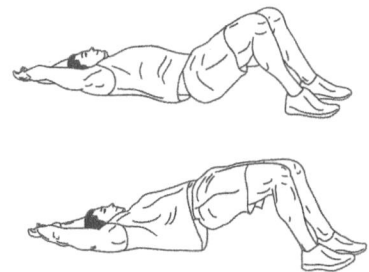

5 bridges

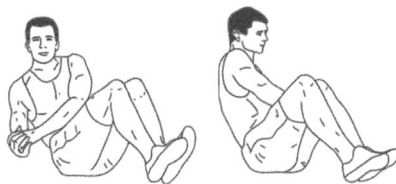

10 sitting twists

84 Rogue Build

Become harder to kill with the Rogue Build Workout! Keep your core tight and stabilize your body for push-up shoulder taps and shoulder taps - placing your feet further apart can help with that. Keep your arms up when performing punches and guard your chin.

Focus: Combat

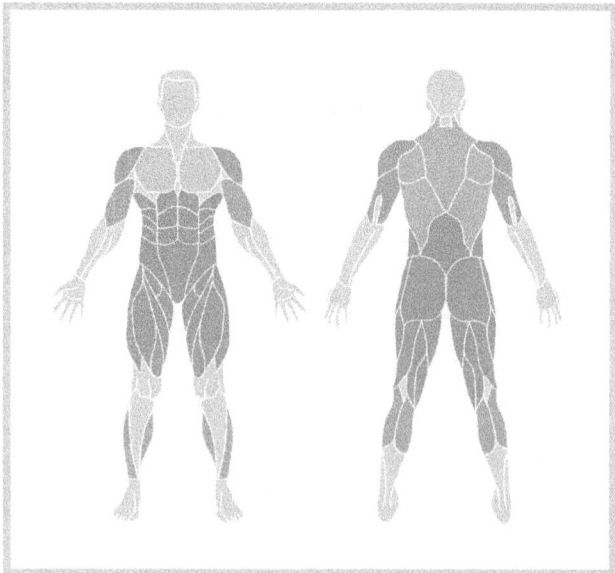

ROGUE BUILD

DAREBEE WORKOUT © darebee.com

LEVEL I 3 sets **LEVEL II** 5 sets **LEVEL III** 7 sets **REST** up to 2 minutes

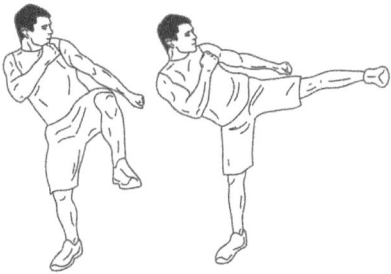

20 side kicks   **10** push-up shoulder taps   **20** side kicks

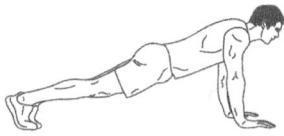

10 shoulder taps   **10-count** plank hold   **10** shoulder taps

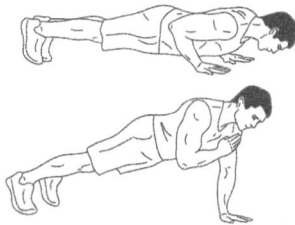

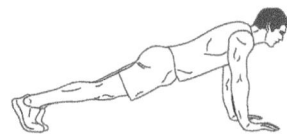

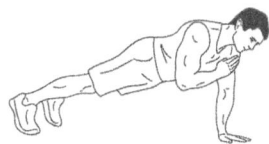

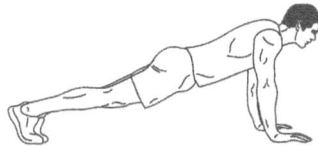

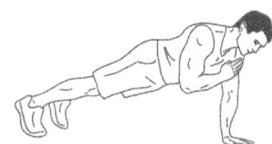

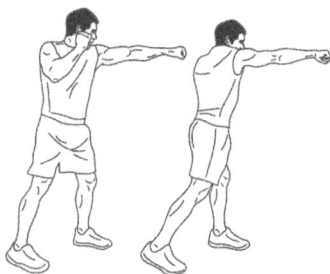

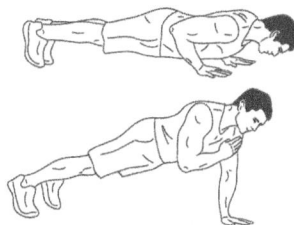

20 punches   **10** push-up shoulder taps   **20** punches

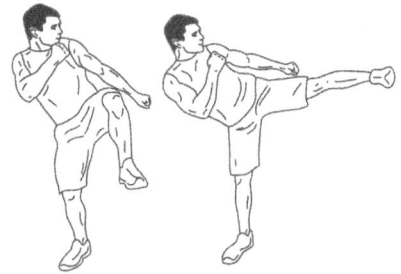

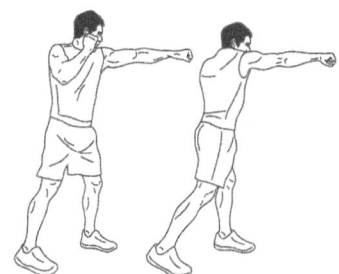

85 Siren

Work on your cardio, balance and coordination with the Siren Workout.
Focus on form and on controlling your breathing throughout the circuit.
Once you've done jumping jacks, try to to take even, deep breaths as you
do the exercises that come afterwards. Finally, when performing side leg
raises raise your leg past your waist and change sides with every repetition.

Focus: High Burn

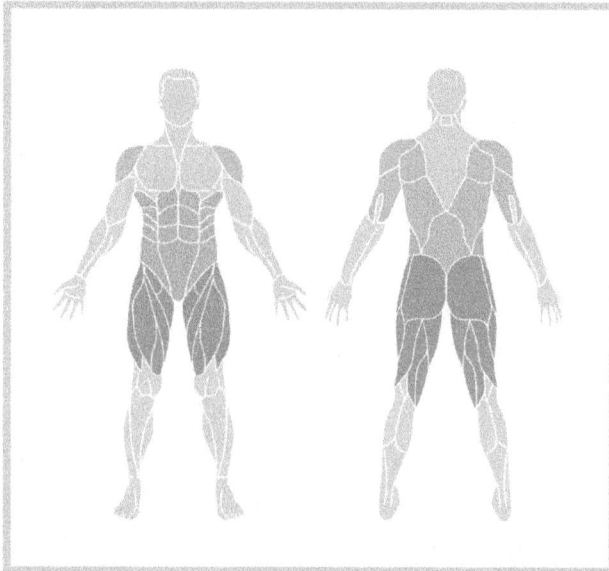

SIREN

DAREBEE WORKOUT © darebee.com

LEVEL I 3 sets LEVEL II 5 sets LEVEL III 7 sets REST up to 2 minutes

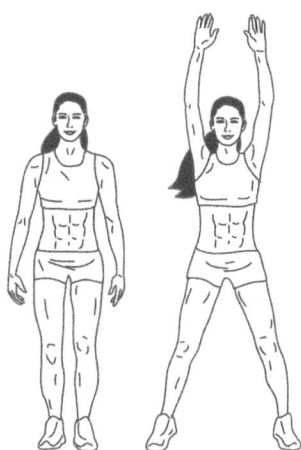

20 jumping jacks   **20** side leg raises   **20-count** balance hold

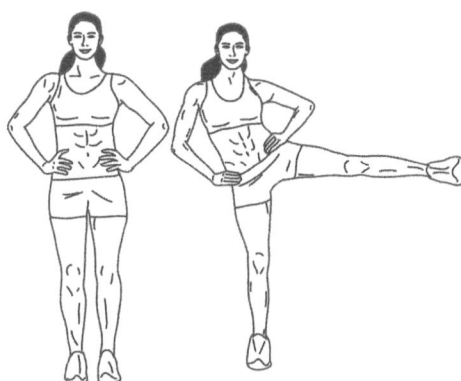

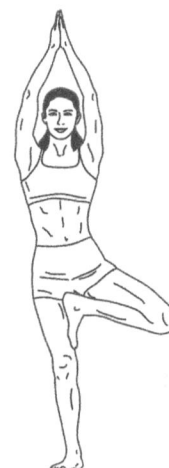

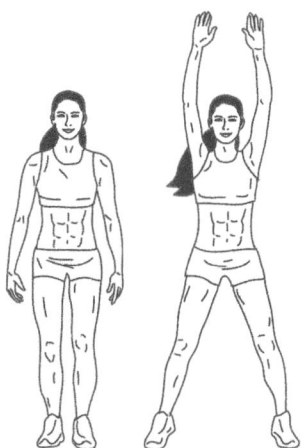

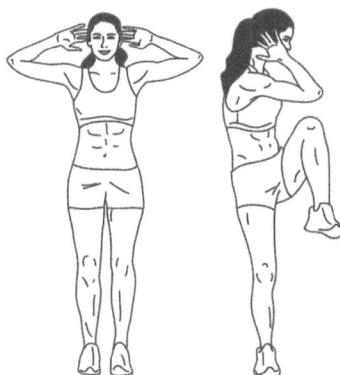

20 jumping jacks   **20** knee-to-elbows   **20-count** balance hold

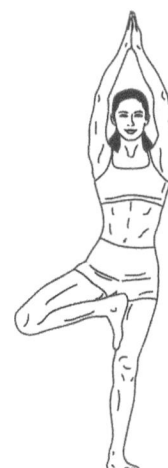

86   Skybreaker

Unleash the power within and reach for the sky with the Skybreaker Workout! Fun but effective combo moves will work your entire body and recruit multiple muscle groups allowing you to reap the full spectrum of bodyweight training benefits. Let your body flow with this routine, mind your form but don't forget to enjoy the process!

Focus: Combat

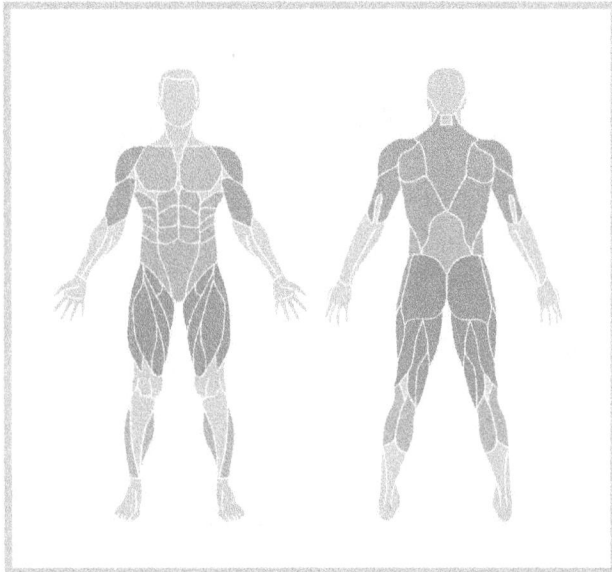

Skybreaker

DAREBEE WORKOUT © darebee.com

LEVEL I 3 sets **LEVEL II** 5 sets **LEVEL III** 7 sets **REST** up to 2 minutes

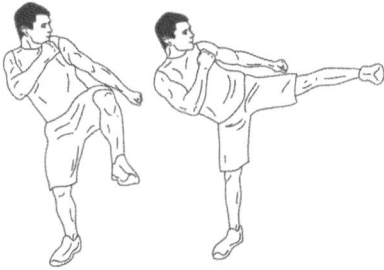

20 side kicks   **20** overhead punches   **20** side kicks

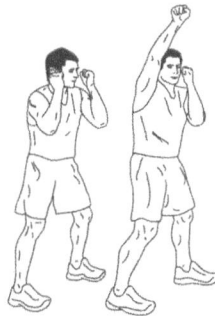

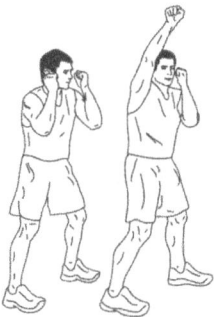

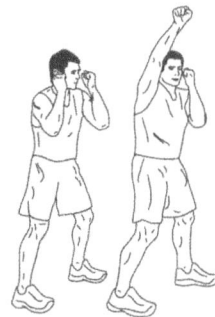

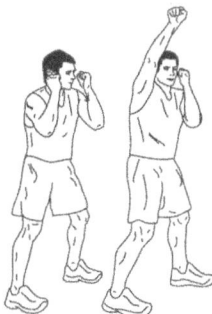

20 overhead punches   **20** backfists   **20** overhead punches

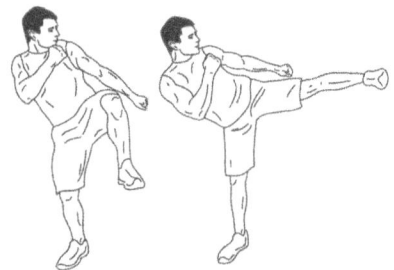

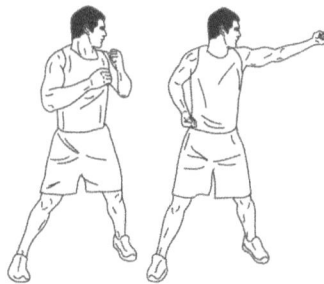

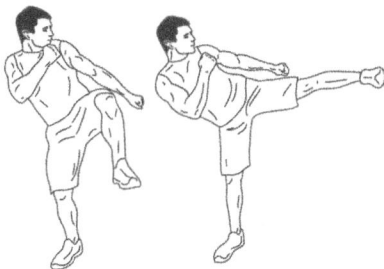

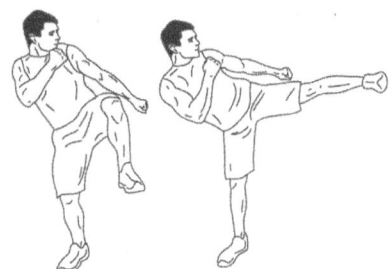

20 side kicks   **20** overhead punches   **20** side kicks

87   Storm

Work your cardio and upper body at the same time with the Storm Workout. Keep your arms up throughout the top sequence and go flat out when doing jumping jacks to get the most out of this routine.

Focus: High Burn

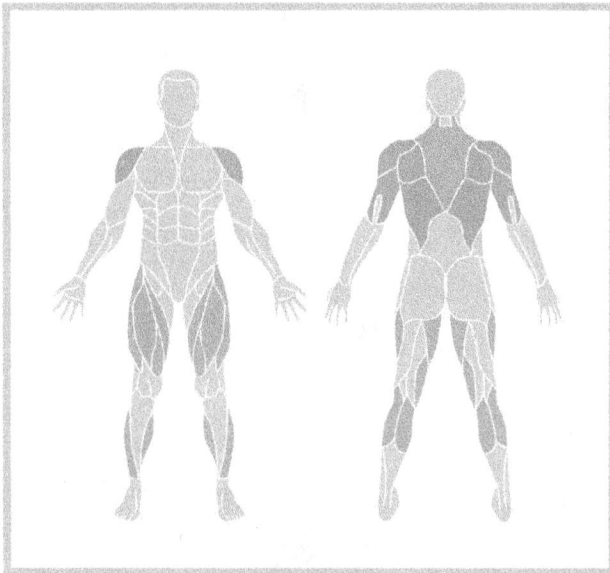

I AM THE STORM

DAREBEE WORKOUT © darebee.com

Level I 3 sets **Level II** 5 sets **Level III** 7 sets | 2 minutes rest

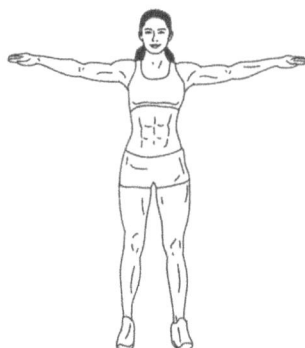

20sec raised arms hold

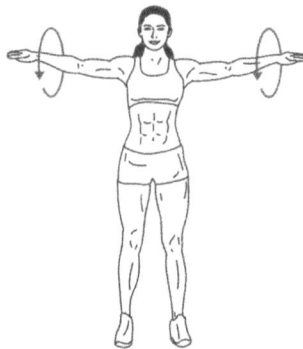

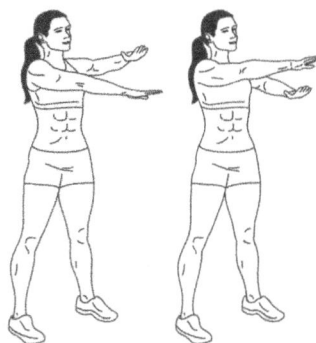

20sec raised arm circles

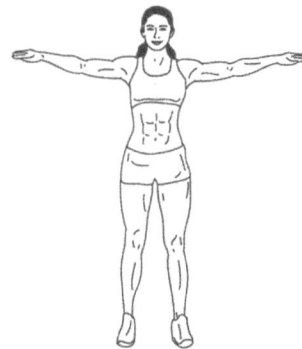

20sec raised arms hold

20sec arm scissors

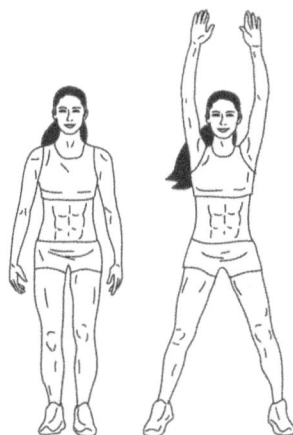

20sec jumping jacks

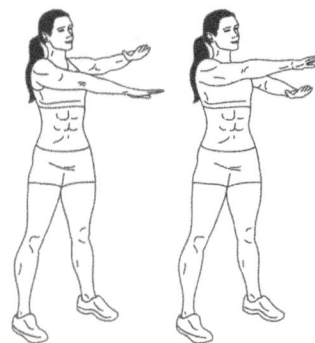

20sec arm scissors

88 Strongman

The numbers count in Strongman as reps build up quickly and body temperature rises. This is a difficulty Level IV workout that helps build up muscle strength and resistance to fatigue. It targets the entire body and helps build up supporting muscle groups that aren't often targeted. It is a transformative workout. All you have to do is make it to the other side of it.

Focus: Strength & Tone

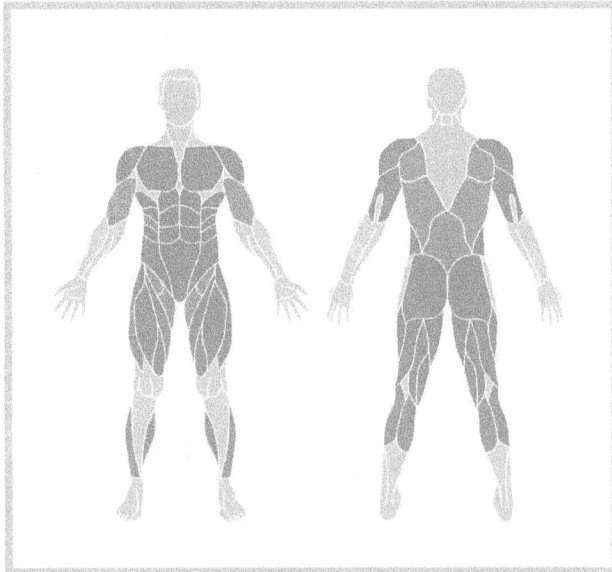

STRONGMAN

DAREBEE WORKOUT © darebee.com

LEVEL I 3 sets **LEVEL II** 5 sets **LEVEL III** 7 sets **REST** up to 2 minutes

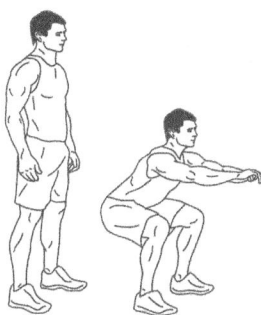

20 squats

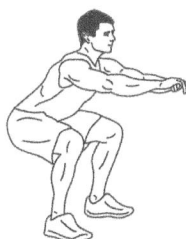

20-count squat hold

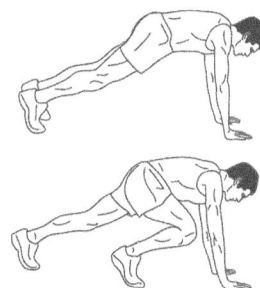

20 slow climbers

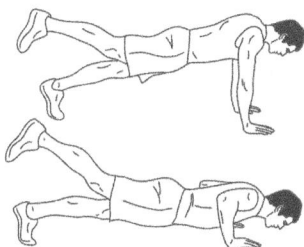

20 raised leg push-ups

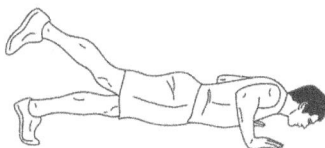

20-count push-up hold

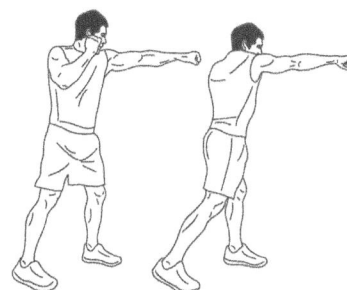

20 punches

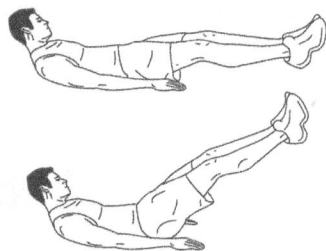

20 leg raises

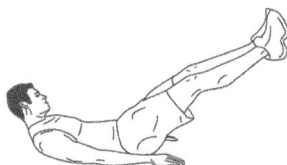

20-count raised leg hold

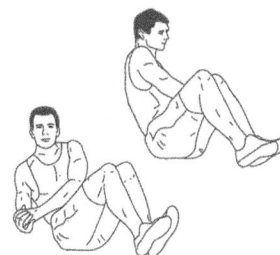

20 sitting twists

89 Super Burn

Get your body into the Super Burn zone with this workout for guaranteed super sweat! Go as fast as you can and try to hit the same number of reps every time you complete each exercise. Keep your arms up throughout the second row of exercises for Extra Credit and aim for a minimum of 10 basic burpees (no push-up) per 20 seconds each time to get the most out of this routine. Catch your breath and repeat!

Focus: High Burn

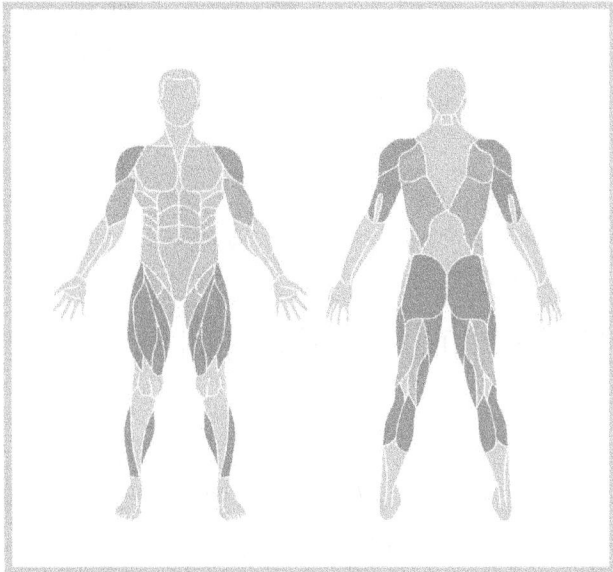

SUPER BURN

DAREBEE HIIT WORKOUT © darebee.com

Level I 3 sets Level II 5 sets Level III 7 sets | 2 minutes rest

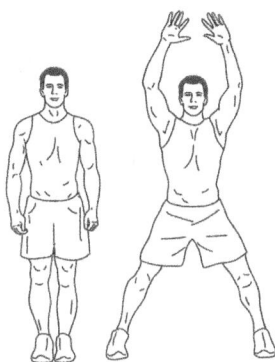

20sec jumping jacks

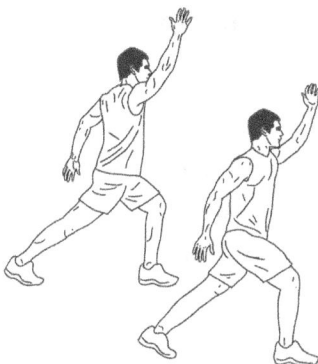

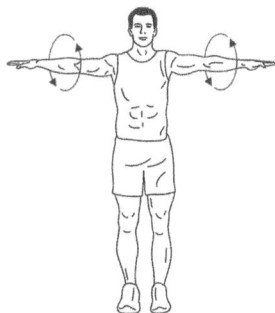

20sec split jacks

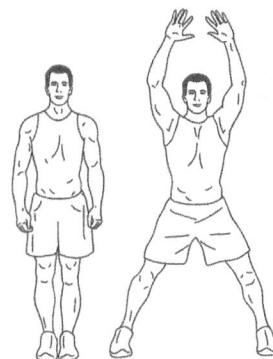

20sec jumping jacks

20sec arm circles

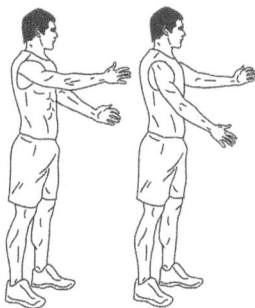

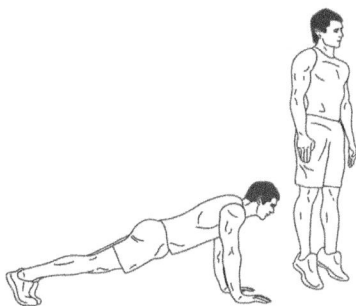

20sec scissor chops

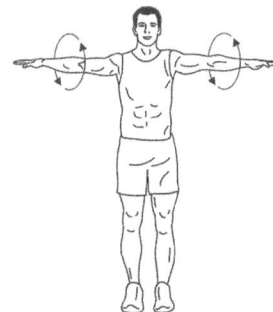

20sec arm circles

20sec basic burpees

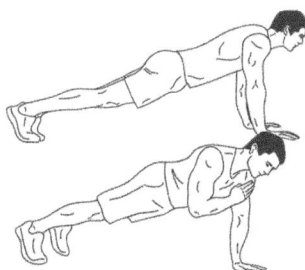

20sec shoulder taps

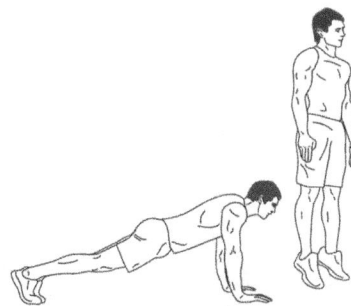

20sec basic burpees

90   Superhero Abs

Superheroes battle evil and fight for good and it's almost a full-time job, but in their spare time they work on their abs (com'on you must have noticed!). To sport the kind of rippling, taut ab wall look that just pops when dressed in spandex, you need the Superhero Abs workout. This is a difficulty Level IV workout so beginners needn't apply (then again Superhero ranks never pull straight from beginners). Make this part of your regular workouts - think at least once a week, maybe more.

Focus: Abs

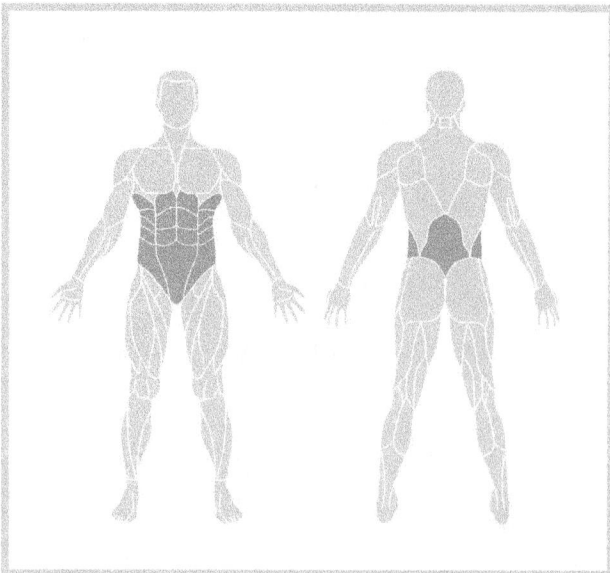

superhero abs

DAREBEE WORKOUT © darebee.com

60 seconds rest between exercises

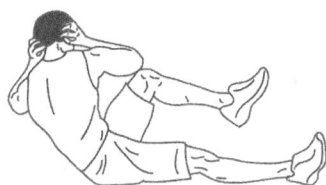

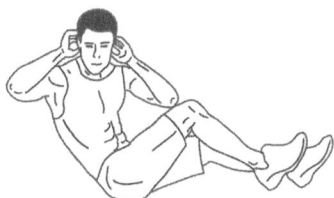

20 knee-to-elbow crunches **x 4 sets**
20 seconds rest between sets

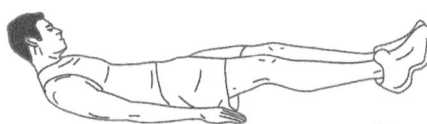

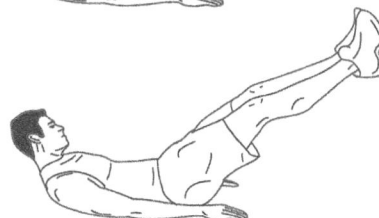

20 leg raises **x 4 sets**
20 seconds rest between sets

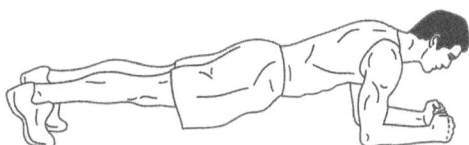

2 minutes elbow plank hold
repeat once

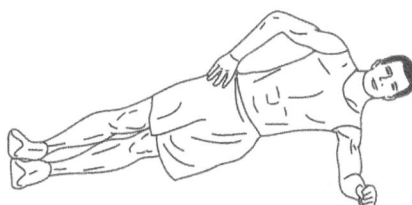

2 minutes side elbow plank
one minute per side | repeat once

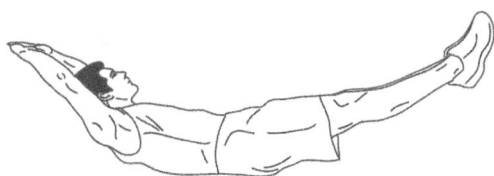

2 minutes hollow hold
repeat once

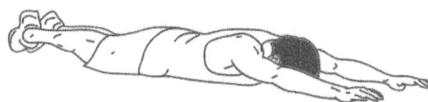

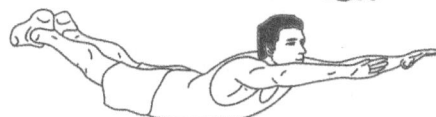

10 superman stretches **x 4 sets**
20 seconds rest between sets

91   Super HIIT

Every now and then you really feel like a "reset" HIIT session, the kind of session that will superheat your muscles, make you sweat hard and leave you feeling totally wiped out afterwards. There are good reasons for sessions like that and they have to do with levelling up. Bring your knees waist high during High Knees, sync your arms and legs, and try to get in as many reps as possible in each 20-second segment. Even done once a month this particular HIIT workout will deliver tangible benefits in overall physical performance.

Focus: High Burn

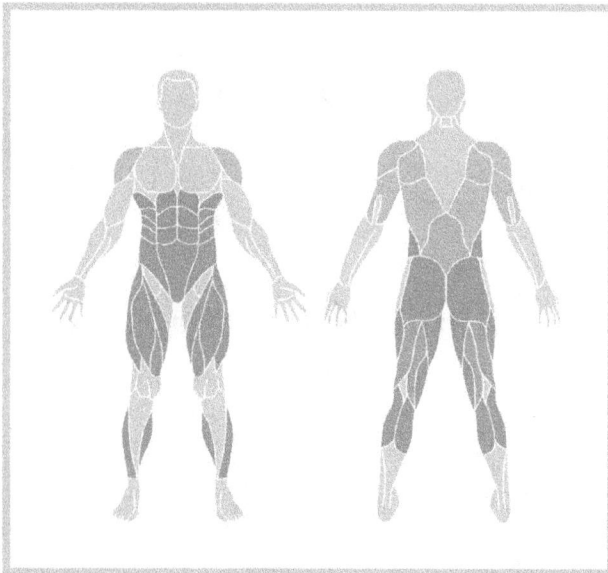

SUPER HIIT

DAREBEE WORKOUT © darebee.com

Level I 3 sets **Level II** 5 sets **Level III** 7 sets | 2 minutes rest

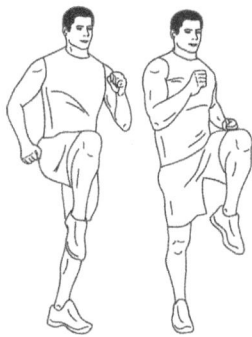

20sec high knees

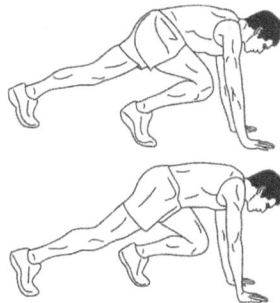

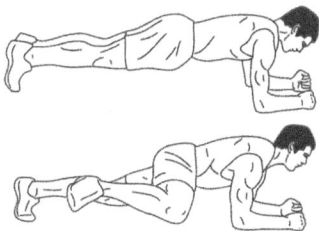

20sec climbers

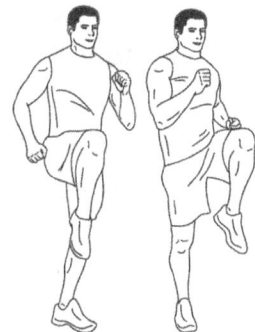

20sec high knees

20sec plank crunches

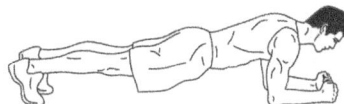

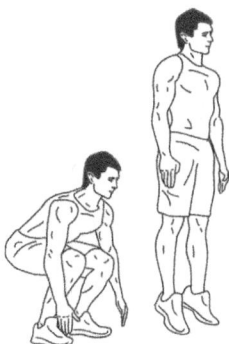

20sec plank hold

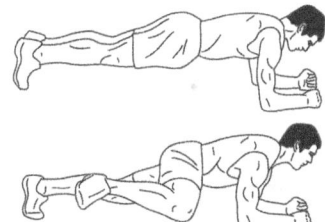

20sec plank crunches

20sec jump squats

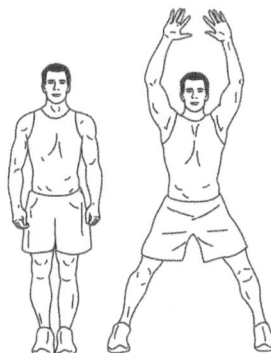

20sec jumping jacks

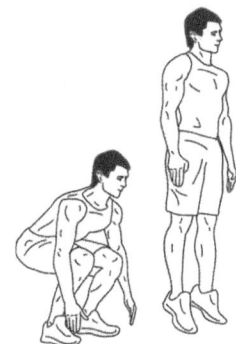

20sec jump squats

92 Superhuman

If you've been a diehard Darebee fan from the very first day and have managed to do each one of our 999 workouts while balancing work, life and sanity we bow before you because you are, by now, truly superhuman, which means you're truly deserving of our 1000th offering. The Superhuman workout hyperloads almost every muscle in your body and then demands extra work from those tendons that power your supportive muscle groups and posture.

Focus: High Burn

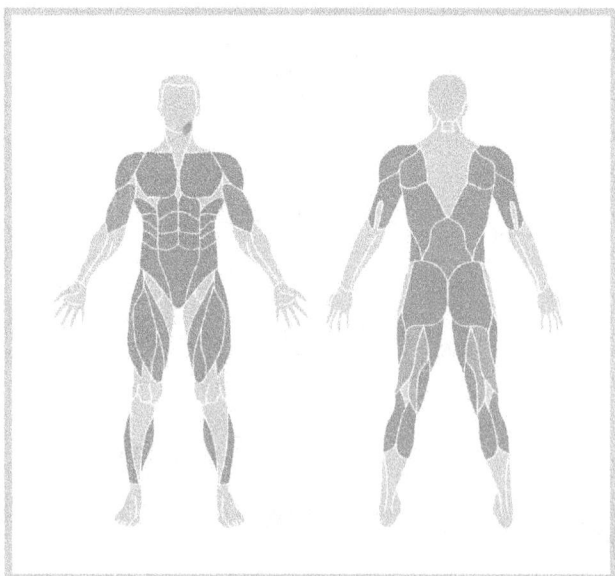

SUPERHUMAN

DAREBEE WORKOUT © darebee.com

LEVEL I 3 sets **LEVEL II** 5 sets **LEVEL III** 7 sets **REST** up to 2 minutes

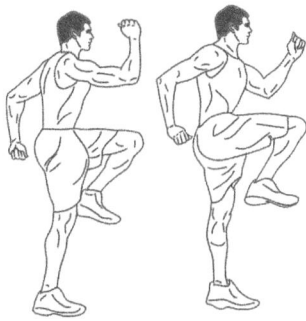

40 march steps

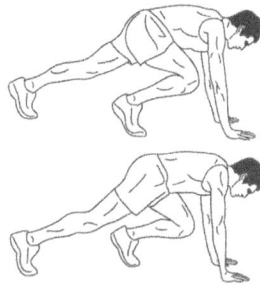

40 climbers

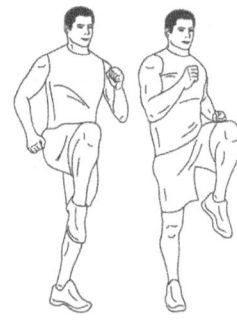

80 high knees

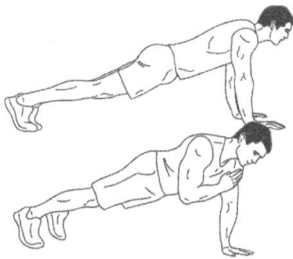

20 shoulder taps

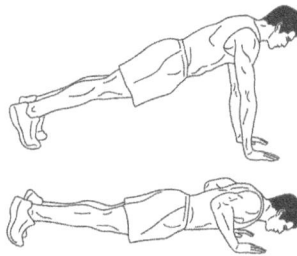

20 push-ups

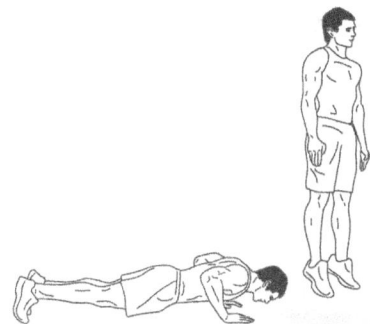

20 burpees

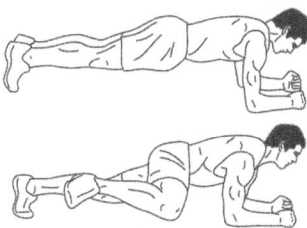

40 plank crunches

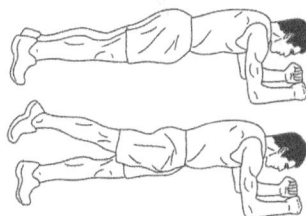

40 plank leg raises

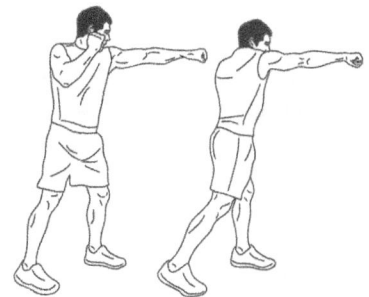

80 punches

93 Sweat Zone

Sweat Zone totally lives up to its name by using all of the body's major muscle groups in strong, dynamic movements and, in the process, utilizing a number of satellite muscle groups. This is a difficulty Level IV workout so you have been warned.

Focus: High Burn

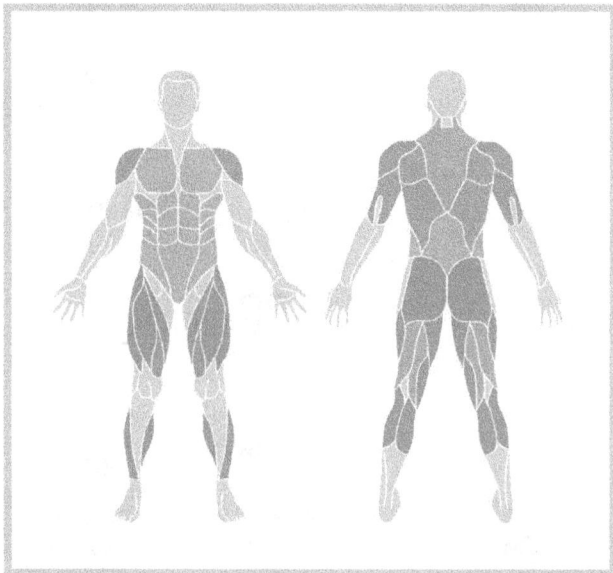

SWEAT ZONE

DAREBEE HIIT WORKOUT © darebee.com

Level I 3 sets **Level II** 5 sets **Level III** 7 sets | 2 minutes rest

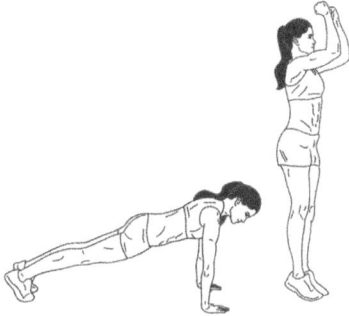

20sec basic burpees **20sec** jumping jacks **20sec** basic burpees

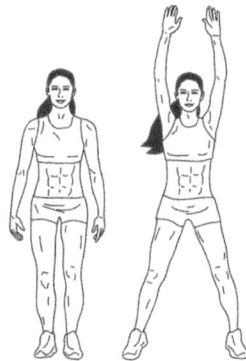

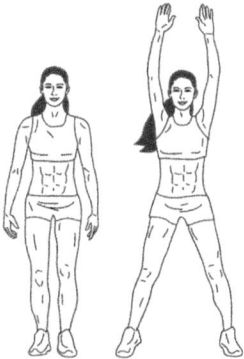

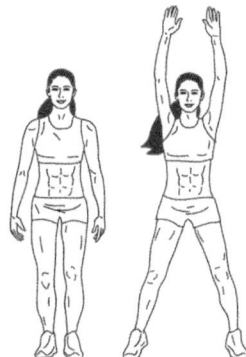

20sec jumping jacks **20sec** side jacks **20sec** jumping jacks

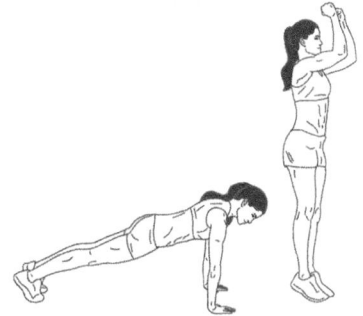

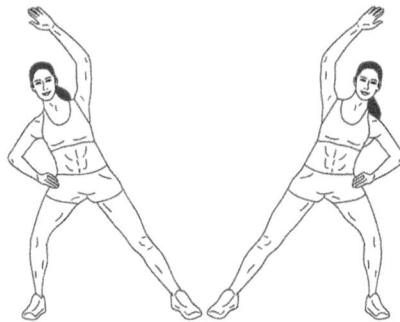

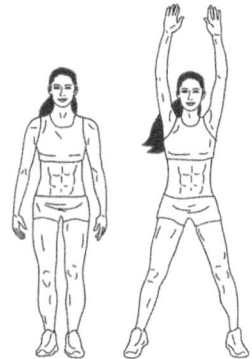

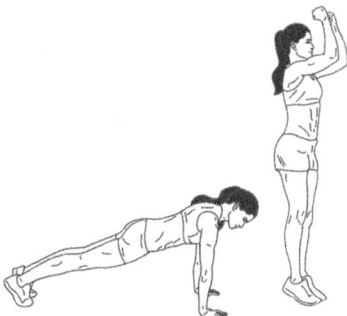

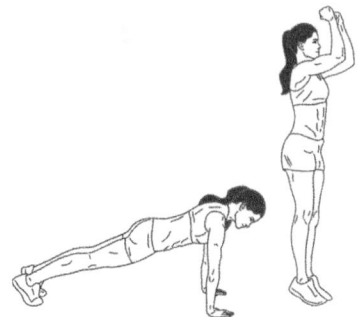

20sec basic burpees **20sec** jumping jacks **20sec** basic burpees

94 Target Abs

Abs are more than just the ripped six-pack look. Strong abs help the body perform faster, with more power. They help maintain better posture, resist fatigue, amplify the transfer of strength from the upper to the lower body and vice versa and they support the lower back and spine better. As the name suggests Target: Abs is a workout that targets the abs. You know what you need to do.

Focus: Abs

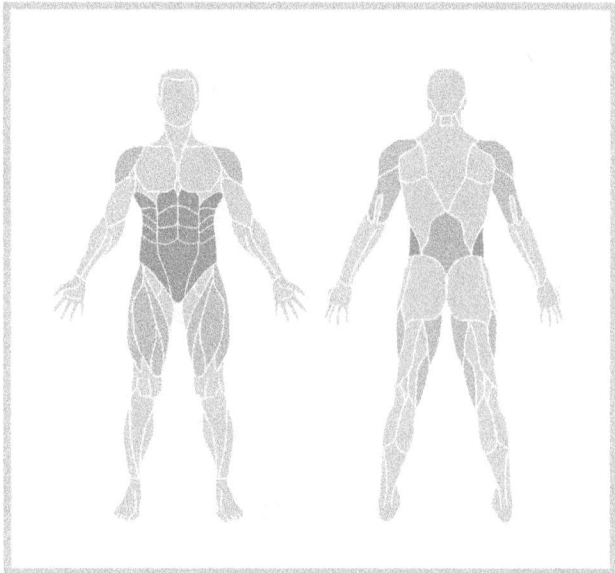

target:abs

DAREBEE WORKOUT © darebee.com

30 seconds each exercise **3 sets in total**

60 seconds rest between sets

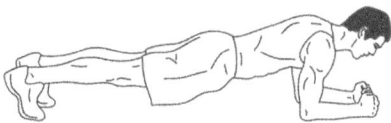

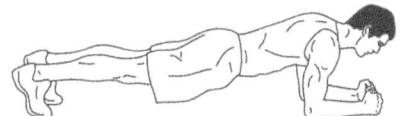

elbow plank hold

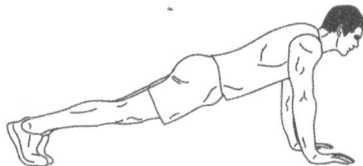

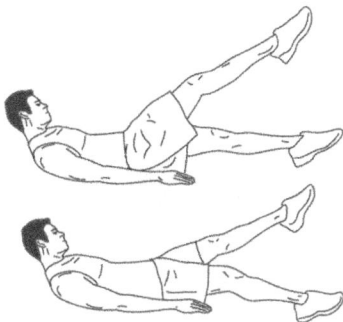

plank hold

elbow plank hold

flutter kicks

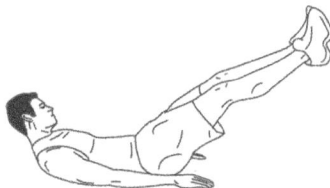

raised legs hold

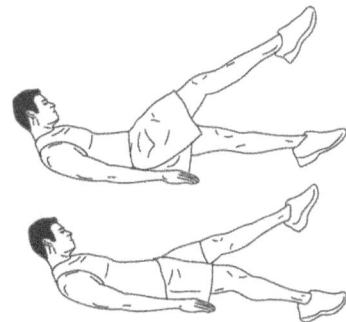

flutter kicks

95 Ultimatum

Combat moves and the conditioning exercises that go with them never make for an "easy" workout which means that if it's easy you want then this ain't the workout you're looking for. The Ultimatum takes you through one exercise after another, adding load upon load until your body aches and your abs shout "enough!". Don't listen to them. Go to the very end and do not stop.

Focus: Strength & Tone

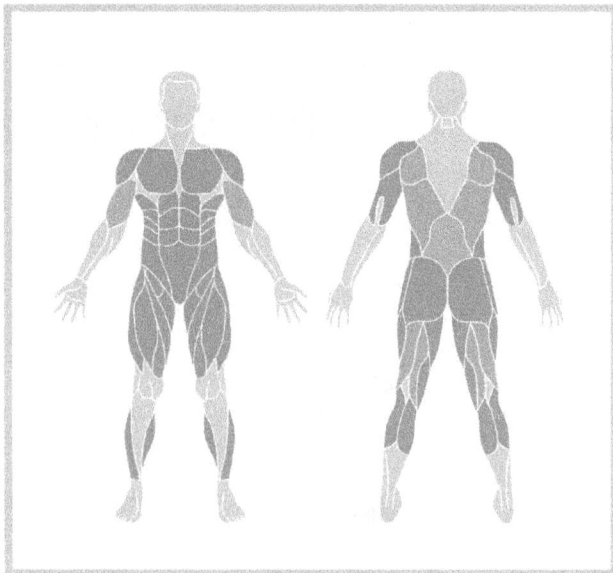

THE *ultimatum*

DAREBEE WORKOUT © darebee.com

LEVEL I 3 sets **LEVEL II** 5 sets **LEVEL III** 7 sets **REST** up to 2 minutes

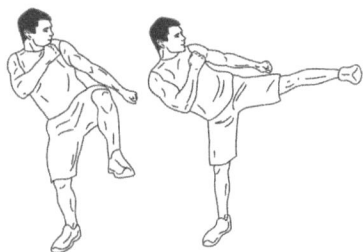

40 side kicks

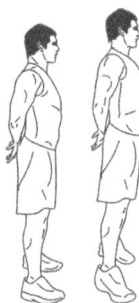

20 calf raises

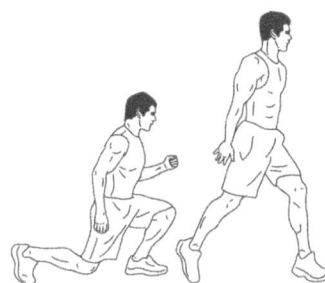

20 jumping lunges

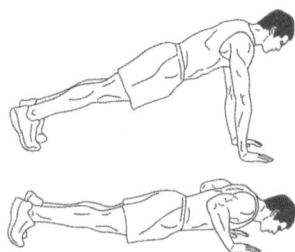

20 push-ups

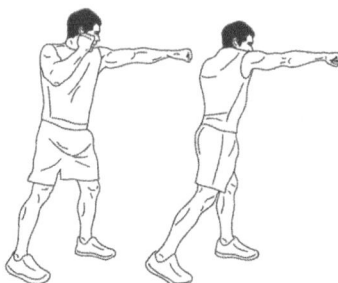

40 punches

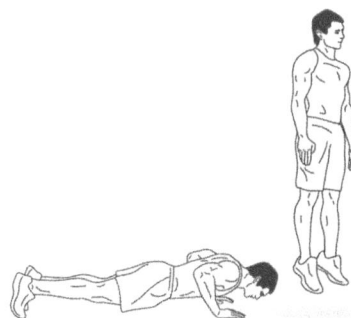

20 burpees

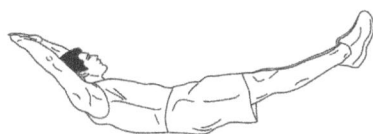

20sec hollow hold

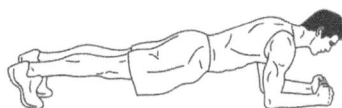

20sec elbow plank

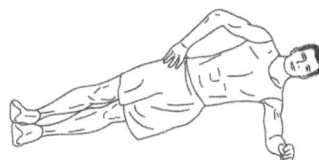

40sec side plank

96 Upperbody Tendons

The Upper Body Tendon Strength workout will help you develop speed and power in your upper body movements. This is not a heavy workout so it should be one you get to do as frequently as possible in order to achieve the necessary structural changes in the tendons.

Focus: Strength & Tone

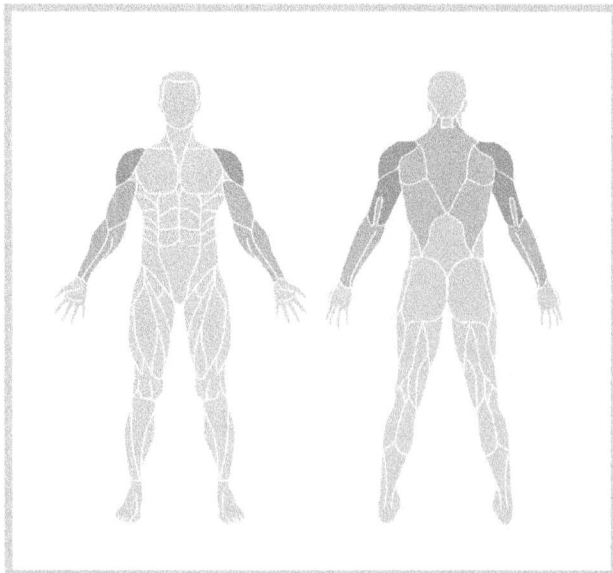

UPPERBODY
TENDON STRENGTH

DAREBEE WORKOUT © darebee.com

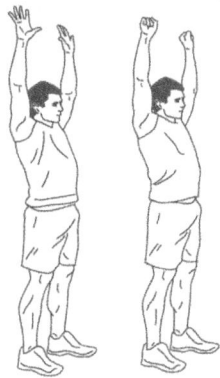

30sec clench/unclench overhead

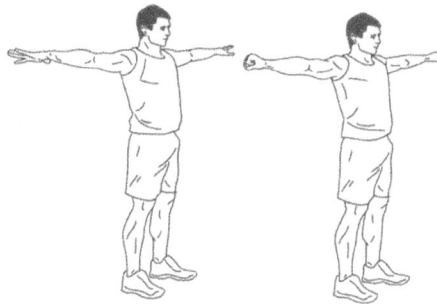

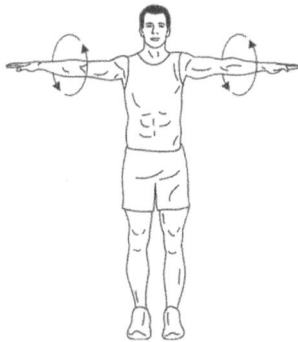

60sec clench / unclench arms raised to the side

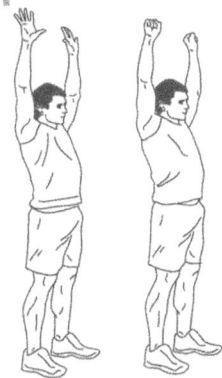

30sec clench/unclench overhead

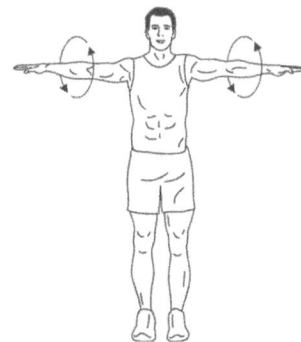

30sec raised arm circles

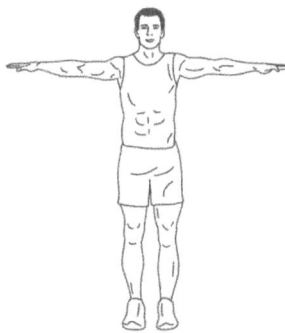

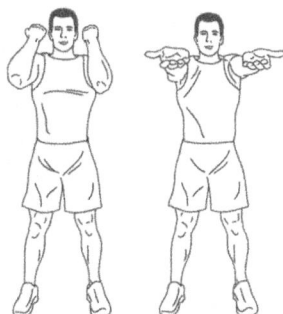

60sec hold

30sec raised arm circles

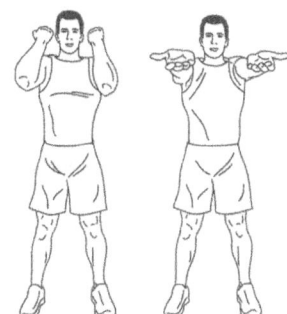

30sec bicep extensions

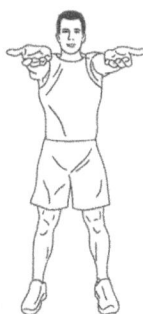

60sec hold

30sec bicep extensions

Upperbody Works

Focus on form rather than speed. When performing bicep extensions, make sure your elbows are pointed forward - don't drop them down. Find your rhythm and stay with it throughout the circuit. Extend your arms all the way during bicep extensions and standing shoulder taps. Once the tensions builds up, you will know it is working.

Focus: Strength & Tone

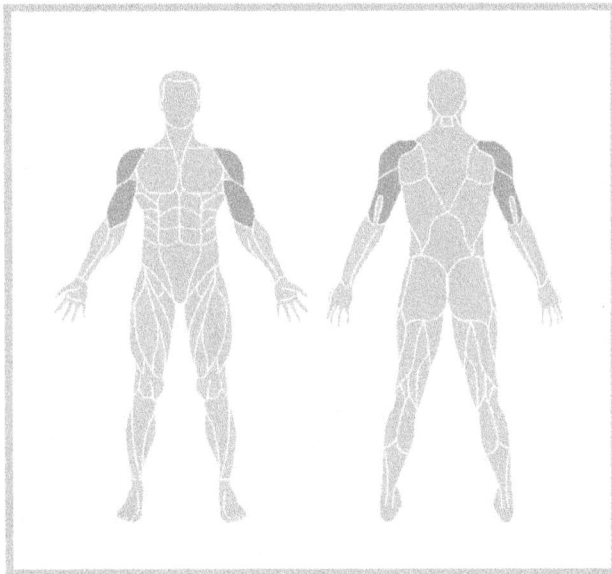

upperbody
works

DAREBEE WORKOUT © darebee.com

LEVEL I 3 sets **LEVEL II** 4 sets **LEVEL III** 5 sets **REST** up to 2 minutes

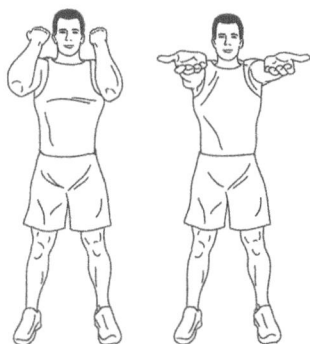

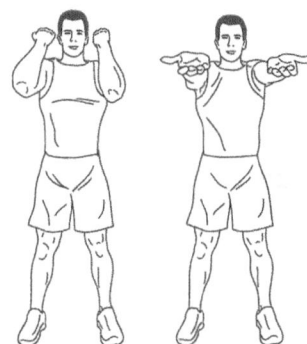

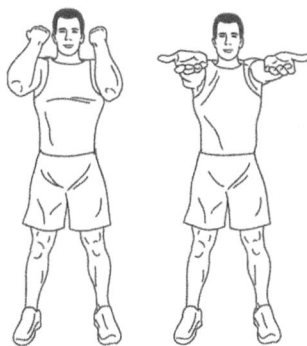

20 bicep extensions   **20** standing shoulder taps   **20** bicep extensions

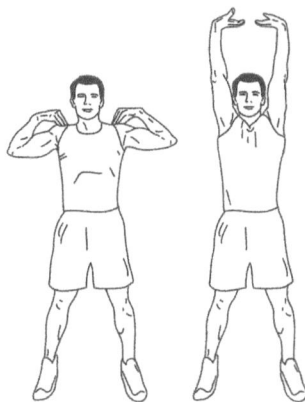

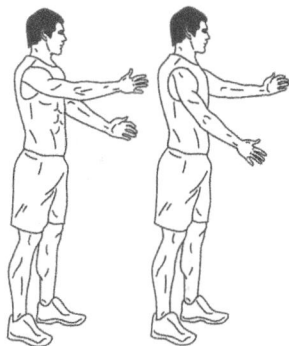

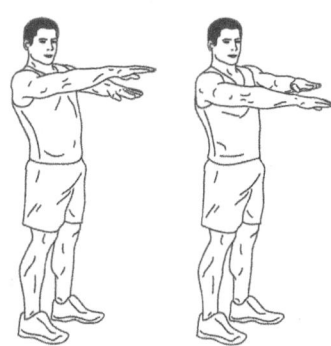

20 scissors chops   **20** bicep extensions   **20** arm scissors

98   Walk, Run, Repeat

We were made to walk and we were made to run. This means our body loves it when we work out the muscles that allow us to walk and run which is why Walk, Run Repeat is a workout that will make you feel good after you've finished.

Focus: High Burn

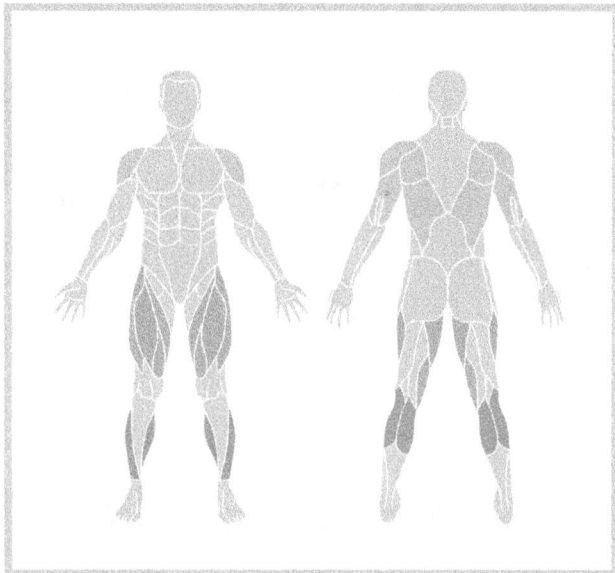

HIIT WORKOUT
BY DAREBEE
© darebee.com

Level I 3 sets
Level II 5 sets
Level III 7 sets
2 minutes rest

WALK
RUN
REPEAT

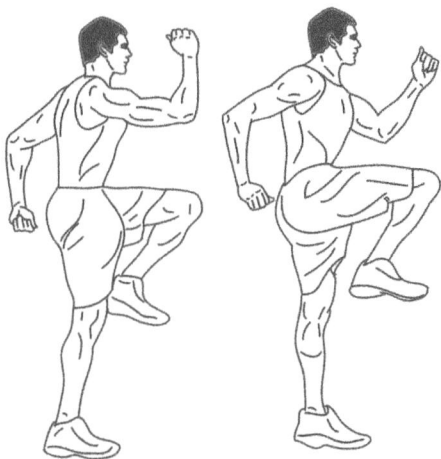

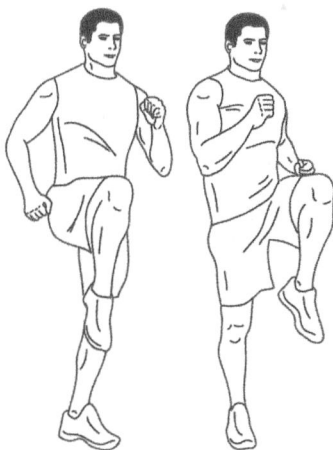

20 sec	march steps
10 sec	high knees
20 sec	march steps
10 sec	high knees
20 sec	march steps
10 sec	high knees
20 sec	march steps
10 sec	high knees
	rest

99 White Rabbit

Agility, flexibility and dexterity are a combination of body and mind. Your body will move well only when your mind has the necessary internal modelling to guide it. The White Rabbit workout helps you develop all of that which means you get to build up all those physical skills necessary for better body control.

Focus: High Burn

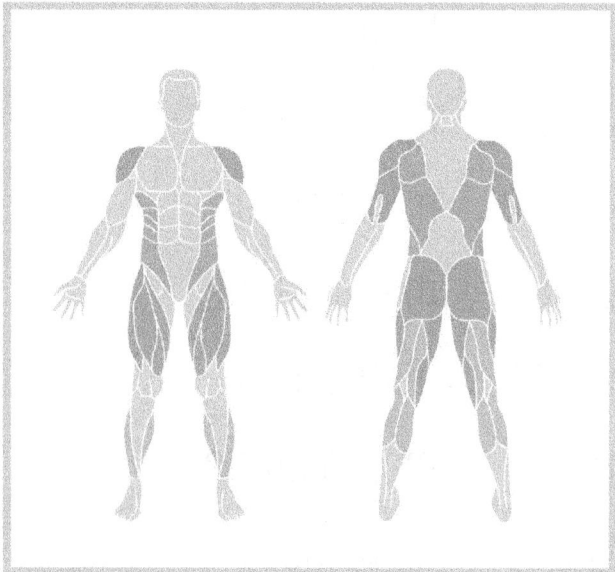

white rabbit

DAREBEE WORKOUT © darebee.com
5 sets in total | 2 minutes rest between sets

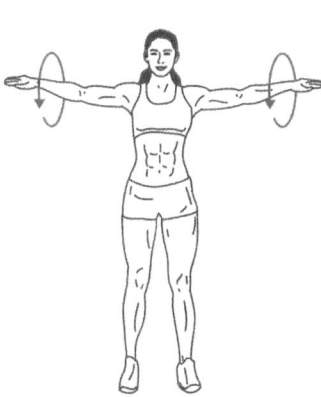

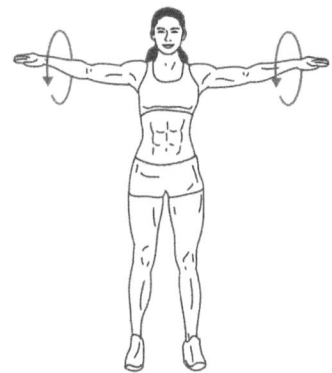

20 raised arm circles

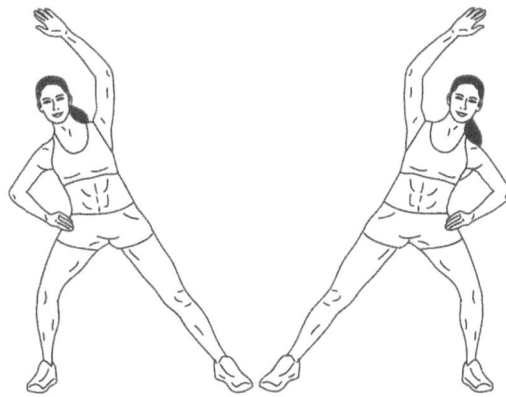

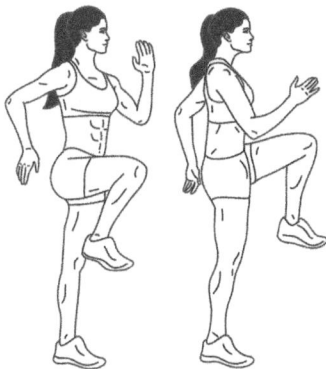

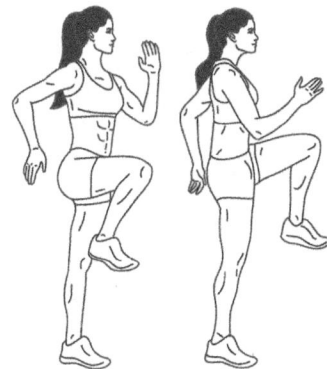

20 side jacks

20 raised arm circles

20 march steps

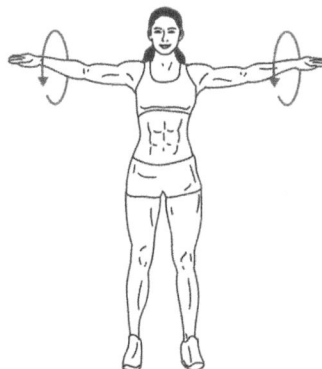

20 raised arm circles

20 march steps

100 Zone

The Zone workout is our classic HIIT with just the right amount of burn to get you sweating but not enough to knock you out (it includes active breaks). It's perfect if you are looking to hit your abs and core and get your lungs a good run for their money. Classic, simple and to the point.

Focus: High Burn

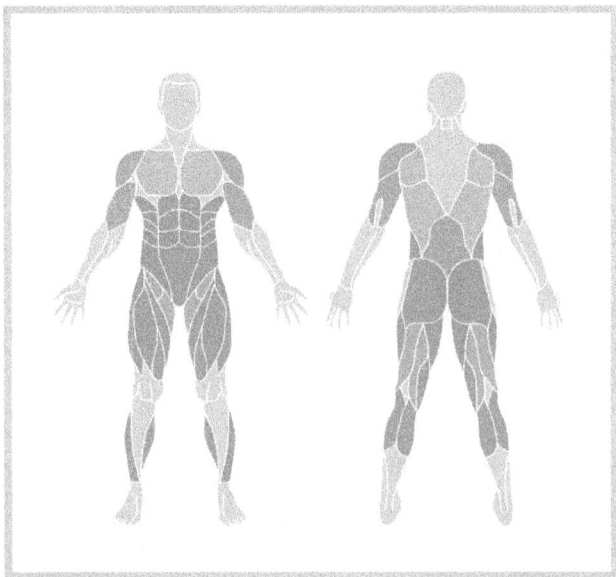

THE ZONE

DAREBEE HIIT WORKOUT © darebee.com

Level I 3 sets **Level II** 5 sets **Level III** 7 sets | 2 minutes rest

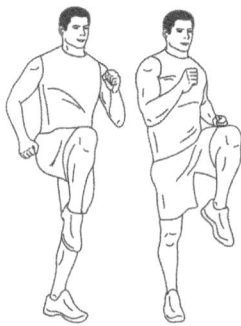

20sec high knees

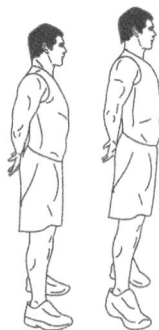

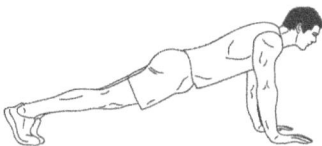

20sec calf raises

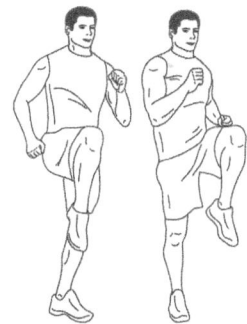

20sec high knees

20sec plank hold

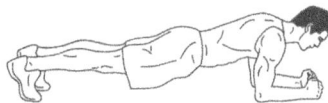

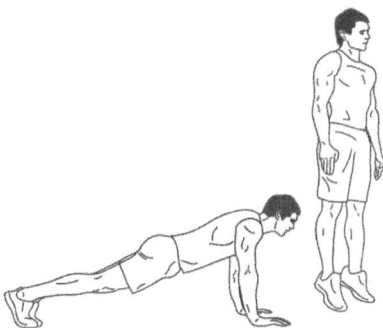

20sec elbow plank hold

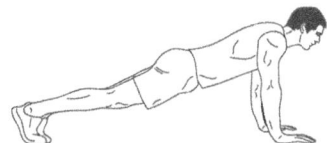

20sec plank hold

20sec basic burpees

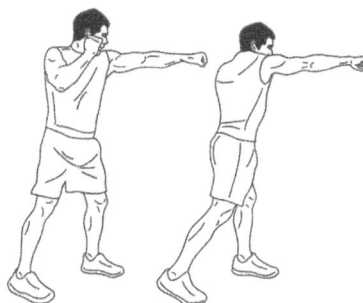

20sec punches

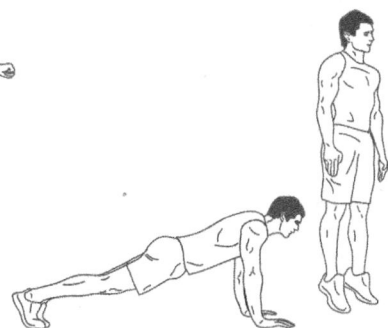

20sec basic burpees

Thank you!

Thank you for purchasing **100 No-Equipment Workouts Vol. 3**, DAREBEE project print edition. DAREBEE is a non-profit global fitness resource dedicated to making fitness accessible for everyone, no matter their circumstances. The project is supported exclusively via user donations and paperback royalties.

After printing costs and store fees every book developed by the DAREBEE project makes $1 and it goes directly into our project maintenance and development fund.

Each sale helps us keep the DAREBEE resource growing, maintain it and keep it up. Thank you for making a difference in its future!

Other books in this series include:

100 No-Equipment Workouts Vol 1.
100 No-Equipment Workouts Vol 2.
100 Office Workouts
Pocket Workouts: 100 no-equipment workouts
ABS 100 Workouts: Visual Easy-To-Follow ABS Exercise Routines for All Fitness Levels

Blank page

www.ingramcontent.com/pod-product-compliance
Lightning Source LLC
Chambersburg PA
CBHW080844270326
41930CB00013B/3000

* 9 7 8 1 8 4 4 8 1 0 1 4 7 *